# SECOND TRIMESTER PREGNANCY TERMINATION

# BOERHAAVE SERIES
# FOR POSTGRADUATE
# MEDICAL EDUCATION
## Vol. 22

BASED ON BOERHAAVE COURSES
ORGANIZED BY
THE FACULTY OF MEDICINE, UNIVERSITY OF LEIDEN
THE NETHERLANDS

# SECOND TRIMESTER PREGNANCY TERMINATION

*edited by*

**MARC J.N.C. KEIRSE**
*Leiden University Medical Centre*

**JACK BENNEBROEK GRAVENHORST**
*Leiden University Medical Centre*

**DIRK A.F. VAN LITH**
*Centre for Human Reproduction, Leiden*

**MOSTYN P. EMBREY**
*University of Oxford*

1982

LEIDEN UNIVERSITY PRESS
THE HAGUE/BOSTON/LONDON

*Distributors:*

*for the United States and Canada*

Kluwer Boston, Inc.
190 Old Derby Street
Hingham, MA 02043
USA

*for all other countries*

Kluwer Academic Publishers Group
Distribution Center
P.O. Box 322
3300 AH Dordrecht
The Netherlands

**Library of Congress Cataloging in Publication Data**                    CIP

Main entry under title:

Second trimester pregnancy termination.

 (Boerhaave series for postgraduate medical
education ; v. 22)
 Includes index.
 1. Abortion.  2. Pregnancy--Trimester, Second.
I. Keirse, Marc J. N. C.  II. Series.
RG734.S43      618.8'8        81-20755
                              AACR2

ISBN-13 : 978-94-009-7971-0      e-ISBN-13: 978-94-009-7969-7
DOI: 10.1007/ 978-94-009-7969-7

*Copyright © 1982 by Martinus Nijhoff Publishers, The Hague.*
Softcover reprint of the hardcover 1st edition 1982

# CONTENTS

# PREFACE

Views and attitudes towards termination of pregnancy have shown considerable evolution over the past few decades. Along with these changes has come a growing concern to adopt means and methods which could make termination easier, safer and more effective. In this evolution, termination in the second trimester in particular is notable as being responsible for a disproportionate share of the complications and adverse experiences associated with pregnancy termination. Although the almost universal shift towards earlier abortion has reduced the number of second trimester procedures as a percentage of the whole, the problems of interrupting pregnancy in the second trimester remain conspicuous. Delay in either seeking or obtaining abortion is still, in many parts of the world, all too frequent. Additionally, recent developments in the prenatal diagnosis of fetal malformations, alphafetoprotein screening programmes and changes in the pattern of and approaches to intrauterine fetal death now also place greater emphasis on the need for adequate methods of interrupting pregnancy in the second trimester.

Unlike the first trimester in which vacuum aspiration is universally considered to be the method of choice, in the second trimester of pregnancy the clinician is faced with alternatives; one method may be more appropriate than another in a particular circumstance and no single method is unequivocally accepted as best. Neither do second trimester terminations form a neatly defined single category. Indeed, any gynaecologist may well question the applicability of the available alternatives in special cases, such as molar pregnancy or intrauterine death, which do not accumulate in large numbers even in specialized abortion clinics or institutions.

Due to considerable advances in intrauterine diagnosis, the number of indications for pregnancy termination based on fetal pathology has increased and will continue to expand as a proportion of all midtrimester procedures.

There is now a growing need for adequate information on suitable methods for termination of pregnancy in the second trimester, including complications, potential risks and long-term effects. This volume provides that information; it deals at length with the comparative merits of the currently favoured alternative techniques, though it does not expand on methods, such as termination hysterotomy and hysterectomy, which should be superseded by a more appropriate procedure. Consideration is given to the historical, demographic and legal aspects of termination of pregnancy in the second trimester, providing a perspective which may prove fruitful in focusing attention on the overall significance of the second trimester procedure as a major problem in pregnancy termination. Additionally, awareness of the factors responsible for delay in securing abortion and the provision of immediate postabortal contraception are discussed as matters of importance which may help reduce the magnitude of the problem, an effect desired by all.

Our thanks are due to Miss H. Wittenberg for her assistance in the editing of this book.

M.J.N.C. KEIRSE
J. BENNEBROEK GRAVENHORST
D.A.F. VAN LITH
M.P. EMBREY

# CONTRIBUTORS

Amy, J.-J., M.D., Department of Gynaecology, Andrology and Obstetrics, Vrije Universiteit Brussel, Academisch Ziekenhuis, Laarbeeklaan 101, B-1090 Brussels, Belgium

Beekhuizen, W., M.D., Centre for Human Reproduction, Kort Rapenburg 1, 2311 GC Leiden, The Netherlands

Bennebroek Gravenhorst, J., M.D., Department of Obstetrics and Gynaecology, University of Leiden Medical Centre, Rijnsburgerweg 10, 2333 AA Leiden, The Netherlands

Berger, G.S., M.D., 917 West Morgan Street, Raleigh, NC 27603, U.S.A.

Cates, W., Jr., M.D., M.P.H., Abortion Surveillance Branch, Family Planning Evaluation Division, Center for Disease Control, Atlanta, GA 30333, U.S.A.

Craft, I., M.D., F.R.C.O.G., Academic Department of Obstetrics and Gynaecology, The Royal Free Hospital, Pond Street, London NW3 2QG, England

Diggory, P., F.R.C.O.G., F.R.C.S., 10 Campden Hill Square, London W8 7LB, England

Du Plessis, M., M.D., Centre for Human Reproduction, Kort Rapenburg 1, 2311 GC Leiden, The Netherlands

Embrey, M.P., M.D., F.R.C.O.G., Nuffield Department of Obstetrics and Gynaecology, University of Oxford, John Radcliffe Hospital, Headington, Oxford OX3 9DU, England

Grimes, D.A., M.D., Abortion Surveillance Branch, Family Planning Evaluation Division, Center for Disease Control, Atlanta, GA 30333, U.S.A.

Ingemanson, C.A., M.D., Department of Obstetrics and Gynecology, Eskilstuna General Hospital, S-631 88 Eskilstuna, Sweden

Keirse, M.J.N.C., M.D., D.P.H., D. Phil., Department of Obstetrics and Gynaecology, University of Leiden Medical Centre, Rijnsburgerweg 10, 2333 AA Leiden, The Netherlands

Keith, G.L., M.D., Department of Obstetrics and Gynecology, Northwestern University Medical School and the Prentice Women's Hospital and Maternity Center, 333 East Superior Street, Chicago, IL 60611, U.S.A.

Kerenyi, T.D., M.D., Department of Obstetrics and Gynecology, The Mount

Sinai Medical Center and Hospital, 1176 Fifth Avenue, New York, NY 10029, U.S.A.

Ketting, E., Ph. D., National Institute for Social Sexuological Research, Dijnselburgerlaan 1, 3705 LP Zeist, The Netherlands

Rioux, J.E., M.D., M.P.H., Department of Obstetrics and Gynaecology, Centre Hospitalier de l'Université Laval, 2705 Boulevard Laurier, Quebec GIV 4 G2, Canada

Hogue, C.J., Ph. D., Department of Biometry and Behavioral Sciences, University of Arkansas for Medical Sciences, 4301 West Markham, Little Rock, AR 72205, U.S.A.

Schnabel, P., Ph. D., Stimezo Nederland (The Netherlands Abortion Foundation), Box 63565, 2503 JN The Hague, The Netherlands

Tietze, C., M.D., The Population Council, One Dag Hammarskjold Plaza, New York, NY 10017, U.S.A.

Van Hall, E.V., M.D., Department of Obstetrics and Gynaecology, University of Leiden Medical Centre, Rijnsburgerweg 10, 2333 AA Leiden, The Netherlands

Van Lith, D.A.F., M.D., Centre for Human Reproduction, Kort Rapenburg 1, 2311 GC Leiden, The Netherlands

Van Schie, K.J., M.D., Centre for Human Reproduction, Kort Rapenburg 1, 2311 GC Leiden, The Netherlands

Yuzpe, A.A., M.D., M.Sc., Department of Obstetrics and Gynaecology, University of Western Ontario, London, Ontario, Canada

# 1. MIDTRIMESTER ABORTION: A GLOBAL VIEW

CHRISTOPHER TIETZE

Midtrimester abortion is responsible for a disproportionate share of adverse experiences associated with the termination of pregnancy. In the United States, abortions performed at 13 weeks gestation or later accounted for 11% of all legal abortions during 1972–77, for an estimated two-thirds of all major complications, and for 57% of all known fatalities. It is important, therefore, to review the levels and trends of midtrimester abortions throughout the world, the demographic and socioeconomic characteristics of the women obtaining them, and the methods used for their performance.

Our review is of necessity limited to data on legal abortions because no information is available for any country on the timing of illegal and self-induced abortions. Survey data are not reliable sources of information on the timing of illegal abortions, nor are hospital records to be depended on for such data, because the risk of complications requiring medical attention is higher after a late abortion than after an early one.

Unfortunately, duration of pregnancy is not uniformly reported in official statistics on abortion. In some countries, e.g., England and Wales, the notification form used includes an entry for the date of onset of the last menstrual period, and gestation is tabulated in terms of completed weeks. As shown in Table 1, this procedure generates a regular declining pattern of abortions by single weeks of gestation. In Czechoslovakia and Scotland, duration of pregnancy is reported by physicians in terms of weeks that they may interpret as ordinal week, nearest week, or completed week, which for '12 weeks' corresponds to 77–83 days, 81–87 days, or 84–90 days, respectively. Moreover,

*Table 1.* Legal abortion at 10-16 weeks gestation, by single weeks: selected areas and years.

| Weeks of gestation | Czecho-slovakia 1975 | England and Wales 1973 | Scotland 1976 | Sweden 1977 |
|---|---|---|---|---|
| 10 | 15223 | 18419 | 1699 | 5205 |
| 11 | 4987 | 15899 | 510 | 3100 |
| 12 | 8049 | 11682 | 871 | 1431 |
| 13 | 133 | 7331 | 215 | 399 |
| 14 | 208 | 4339 | 361 | 393 |
| 15 | 65 | 2632 | 130 | 303 |
| 16 | 105 | 1828 | 260 | 266 |

*M.J.N.C. Keirse et al. (eds.), Second Trimester Pregnancy Termination. All rights reserved*
*Copyright © 1982 Martinus Nijhoff Publishers, The Hague/Boston/London.*

the reported figures tend to bunch at even numbers of weeks and especially at multiples of four, corresponding to lunar months. As a result of this preference, many abortions performed at 13 weeks of gestation are reported at 12 weeks, thus reducing the number of midtrimester procedures. Sweden, which requires reporting in terms of completed weeks but provides careful instructions defining duration of pregnancy, also has largely avoided the heaping at even numbers of weeks. Finally, while physicians in general follow the tradition of counting the duration of pregnancy from the first day of the last menstrual period, some may count from the estimated day of conception. For all these reasons, information on time trends and group differences within countries is more reliable than comparisons between countries.

The overall frequency of midtrimester legal abortions depends on the applicable law. All countries authorizing abortions on medical or fetal indications permit midtrimester abortions on these grounds, but few countries permit such abortions at the request of the pregnant woman or on social or social-medical indications. As of mid-1979 the latter included some of the states of Australia, Great Britain, Hong Kong, India, Israel, Japan, Singapore, Sweden (up to 18 weeks), the United States, and Zambia [15].

Table 2 shows the percentages of midtrimester abortions among all legal abortions in nine countries and New York City for each year of the 1968–77 decade or for those years for which data were available. A shift towards earlier abortion has occurred in almost all countries shown in the table, most dramatically in Sweden, where midtrimester abortions dropped from 57% in 1968 to 6% in 1977. This trend probably reflects (a) a growing awareness among women and physicians that abortion is safer early in pregnancy than later on, and (b) the increasing availability of abortion services. Exceptions to the general trend toward earlier abortions were recorded for Czechoslovakia and Hungary, where the proportions of midtrimester abortions rose when access to abortion on request — but not to abortion on medical grounds — was restricted.

In recent years the proportion of midtrimester abortions by country was highest in India (averaging 24% for 1972-75), followed in descending order by a cluster consisting of Scotland, Canada and residents of England and Wales (16–18%), with comparable figures for the United States, Sweden, and Japan ranging from 4 to 9%. In Hungary and Czechoslovakia, where midtrimester abortions are generally limited to those performed for medical reasons, the proportion of all midtrimester abortions was less than one per 100 legal abortions.

In New York City, for the years 1973–75, the increased proportions of midtrimester procedures among nonresident women contrast with a downward trend for residents and suggest a selective migration from other areas where first trimester abortions performed in clinics became available more

Table 2. Midtrimester abortions per 100 legal abortions: selected areas, 1968–77.

| Area and characteristic[1] | 1968 | 1969 | 1970 | 1971 | 1972 | 1973 | 1974 | 1975 | 1976 | 1977 |
|---|---|---|---|---|---|---|---|---|---|---|
| Canada [1] | na[2] | na | na | na | na | na | 21.2 | 18.7 | 16.9 | 15.8 |
| Czechoslovakia [3] | 0.5 | 0.5 | 0.5 | 0.5 | 0.6 | 0.6 | 0.5 | 0.4 | 0.5 | 0.8 |
| England and Wales [16, 17] | | | | | | | | | | |
| Residents | 38.0 | 34.3 | 28.7 | 23.3 | 20.4 | 18.1 | 17.2 | 17.4 | 16.5 | 16.4 |
| Nonresidents | 36.3 | 38.1 | 26.9 | 21.6 | 18.9 | 22.7 | 25.6 | 28.5 | 32.0 | 32.0 |
| Hungary [6, 7] | na | na | na | 0.5 | 0.5 | 0.5 | 1.0 | 0.8 | 0.7 | 0.8 |
| India [8] | na | na | na | na | na | na | nearly 24 | — | na | na |
| Japan [9][3] | 5.0 | 4.8 | 4.5 | 4.1 | 3.8 | 3.4 | 3.2 | 3.2 | 4.1 | 4.2 |
| New York City [11] | | | | | | | | | | |
| Residents | na | na | na | 20.7 | 16.1 | 15.1 | 14.5 | 11.7 | 9.7 | 9.1 |
| Nonresidents | na | na | na | 18.8 | 18.2 | 25.8 | 25.6 | 24.1 | 19.6 | 22.4 |
| Scotland [18] | na | 35.0 | 28.0 | 25.6 | 20.9 | 19.2 | 16.9 | 18.0 | 17.8 | na |
| Sweden [13] | 57.1 | 49.3 | 40.5 | 32.6 | 26.6 | 19.7 | 13.3 | 7.0 | 6.4 | 6.0 |
| United States[4] | na | na | na | na | 15.3 | 14.5 | 12.0 | 10.8 | 9.7 | 9.0 |

[1] References between parentheses.

[2] Na = not available.

[3] Gestation reported in months. Midtrimester abortions (4 months or more) were 19.2% in 1951 and 13.6% in 1952, dropping gradually to 5.0% in the late 1960s.

[4] Author's estimates based on references [4] and [19].

rapidly than did midtrimester procedures requiring hospitalization. By 1976 the great majority of nonresident women came from nearby suburban areas, thus reducing the selection by duration of pregnancy. In 1977 the trend was reversed, indicating a tightening of hospital policies in other areas and in 1978 the proportion of midtrimester abortions for nonresidents again reached 25.4% (not shown). In that year about 600 *more* women came to New York City to obtain second trimester abortions than in 1976, compared with about 100 000 who were able to obtain these services elsewhere. First-trimester abortions to nonresidents *declined* by 2400 from 1976 to 1978, thus driving up the percentage of midtrimester procedures. A marked increase in the proportion of second trimester abortions among nonresidents also occurred in England beginning in 1974 as first trimester abortion became increasingly available to many European women, first in the Netherlands and later also in their own countries.

Table 3 presents a different approach to the statistics of midtrimester abortions, showing them as a rate per 1000 women, aged 15–44, for selected areas and available years for the 1968–77 decade rather than as a percentage of all legal abortions. Thus computed, the incidence of midtrimester abortion is higher in England and Wales than in Scotland, higher in the United States than in Canada or in England, still higher in Japan, and highest in New York City. The highest midtrimester abortion rate, 16 per 1000 women, 15–44 years of age (not shown in Table 3), has been reported from Seoul, based on a survey of providers of abortion services conducted in 1977–78 [5]. The rapidly declining proportions of second trimester abortions among all legal abortions in Sweden in 1968–72 and in the United States in 1972–77, shown in Table 2, are not reflected in Table 3 because these declines coincided with increases in the overall abortion rate.

Women of low socioeconomic status (Table 4) and especially the youngest women (Table 5) had the highest proportions of late abortions. The strong inverse association of period of gestation and woman's age probably reflects the inexperience of the very young in recognizing the symptoms of pregnancy, their unwillingness to accept the reality of their situation, their ignorance about where to seek advice and help, and their hesitation to confide in adults. Economic considerations and, in many places, regulations prohibiting surgery on minors without parental consent undoubtedly contributed to delays.

The very high proportions of midtrimester abortions, shown in Table 5 for the youngest women, actually understate the situation. For example, a woman who conceives at 14 years and 9 months and has a first trimester abortion will appear in the '14 or less' age group; if she has a midtrimester abortion, she will be in the next higher age group. Since about one-third of all pregnancies initiated before age 15 which were aborted in England and Wales and about one-fourth of comparable pregnancies in the United States in 1977

Table 3. Midtrimester abortions per 1000 women, 15–44: selected areas, 1968–77

| Area | 1968 | 1969 | 1970 | 1971 | 1972 | 1973 | 1974 | 1975 | 1976 | 1977 |
|---|---|---|---|---|---|---|---|---|---|---|
| Canada | na | na | na | na | na | na | 2.0 | 1.8 | 1.7 | 1.7 |
| Czechoslovakia | 0.2 | 0.2 | 0.2 | 0.2 | 0.2 | 0.1 | 0.1 | 0.1 | 0.1 | 0.2 |
| England and Wales[1] | 1.3 | 1.8 | 2.3 | 2.4 | 2.3 | 2.1 | 2.0 | 1.9 | 1.8 | 1.7 |
| Hungary | na | na | na | 0.4 | 0.4 | 0.4 | 0.4 | 0.3 | 0.3 | 0.3 |
| Japan[2] | 5.4 | 5.1 | 4.7 | 4.3 | 3.9 | 3.3 | 3.1 | 3.0 | 3.8 | 3.8 |
| New York City[1] | na | na | na | 8.2 | 6.7 | 7.3 | 7.4 | 5.7 | 4.8 | 4.7 |
| Scotland | na | 1.3 | 1.5 | 1.6 | 1.6 | 1.4 | 1.3 | 1.3 | 1.2 | na |
| Sweden | 4.0 | 4.3 | 4.1 | 4.0 | 4.0 | 3.2 | 2.6 | 1.4 | 1.3 | 1.2 |
| United States | na | na | na | na | 2.0 | 2.4 | 2.4 | 2.4 | 2.4 | 2.3 |

[1] Residents only.
[2] Based on Muramatsu's estimate [10] of actual number of legal abortions in 1970 (2 780 000) and trend of reported abortions 1968–77.

*Table 4.* Midtrimester abortions per 100 legal abortions by occupation group, within marital status: England and Wales, 1968 and 1973.[1]

| Occupation Group | Single women by own occupation | | Married women by husband's occupation | |
|---|---|---|---|---|
| | 1968 | 1973 | 1968 | 1973 |
| Professional | 23.3 | 14.4 | 23.0 | 8.9 |
| Intermediate | 31.7 | 15.0 | 29.1 | 10.3 |
| Skilled | 37.5 | 19.1 | 41.2 | 14.5 |
| Semi-skilled | 41.0 | 23.5 | 42.6 | 16.2 |
| Unskilled | 48.0 | 26.6 | 48.5 | 20.4 |

[1] Residents.

occurred between 14 years and 9 months and 15 years of age, this distortion is by no means negligible although it cannot be quantified.

The slight increases in the proportions of midtrimester procedures, observed in all areas among the oldest women shown in Table 5, reflect primarily the association of high order pregnancies with low socioeconomic status. Abortions on medical grounds are also more common among older women and some women in their forties may have misinterpreted the amenorrhea of pregnancy as the onset of menopause.

The various methods used to terminate pregnancy in midtrimester can be grouped under three general headings: dilatation and evacuation (D&E), hysterotomy and hysterectomy, and medical induction.

As shown in Table 6, dilatation and evacuation by the vaginal route is primarily employed in the early part of the second trimester (13–16 weeks). Its use has increased over the past several years in both the United States and England where it represents the highest proportion for any country, and is particularly high in the private sector compared with the hospitals of the National Health Service (NHS). D & E is substantially less frequently used in Sweden and generally limited to pregnancies of 13 or 14 weeks gestation.

Hysterotomy and hysterectomy, on the other hand, are performed more often in the later than in the earlier part of the second trimester in England and Wales and also in Sweden. Resort to these major surgical procedures has declined dramatically in the United States and especially in England where it had been very high during the period immediately following the implementation of the 1967 Abortion Act. This high level was clearly associated with a strong tendency to perform abortion and sterilization concurrently. In 1977, both abortions by hysterotomy or hysterectomy and surgical sterilizations were performed much more often in NHS-hospitals than in the private sector.

Of all midtrimester abortions by hysterotomy *or* hysterectomy 4% were done by hysterectomy in England and Wales in 1968 and 10% in 1977, and

Table 5  Midtrimester abortions per 100 legal abortions, by woman's age  selected areas and periods

| Area | Period | Woman's age (years) | | | | | | | |
|---|---|---|---|---|---|---|---|---|---|
| | | 14 or less | 15–17 | 18–19 | 20–24 | 25–29 | 30–34 | 35–39 | 40 or more |
| Canada | 1976 | 33 5 | 27 2 | 21 7 | 16 3 | 11 5 | 10 4 | 10 7 | 14 1 |
| England & Wales[1] | 1976 | 30 6 | 23 2 ——— | | 18 2 | 13 8 | 10 6 | 10 0 | 12 3 |
| Hungary | 1977 | 3 3 ——— | | | 0 5 | 0 5 | 0 5 | 0 3 | 0 7 |
| India[2] | 1972–75 | 41 9 ——— | | | 15 6 | 10 8 | 14 0 | 17 0 ——— | |
| Japan | 1977 | 19 1 ——— | | | 8 0 | 4 1 | 2 6 | 2 4 | 2 8 |
| New York City[1] | 1977 | 27 6 | 18 4 | 12 3 | 9 0 | 6 9 | 5 9 | 6 1 | 6 5 |
| Sweden | 1975–76 | 10 6 ——— | | 9 1 | 6 9 | 5 0 | 4 1 | 4 3 | 6 7 |
| United States[3] | 1972–75 | 18 6 ——— | | | 12 2 | 9 9 | 9 7 | 10 0 ——— | |

[1] Residents only
[2] Karnataka State [12]
[3] Distribution by age and gestation estimated by iterative adjustment of a known distribution (JPSA/CDC) to marginal totals for the United States [2]

*Table 6.* Percent distribution of midtrimester abortions by type of procedure, within weeks of gestation: selected areas and periods.

| Area, period, and weeks of gestation | Dilatation and evacuation[1] | Hysterotomy or hysterectomy | Medical induction | Other procedures |
|---|---|---|---|---|
| **Canada, 1977** | | | | |
| 13–16 | 68.9 | 3.8 | 27.3 | na |
| 17 or more | 9.5 | 3.9 | 86.6 | na |
| **England and Wales, 1968[2]** | | | | |
| 13–16 | 50.0 | 42.5 | 7.5 | |
| 17 or more | 16.7 | 68.5 | 14.8 | |
| **England and Wales, 1977[2]** | | | | |
| 13–16 | 77.4 | 2.7 | 19.6 | 0.3 |
| 17 or more | 40.6 | 3.2 | 55.9 | 0.3 |
| **NHS-hospitals, 1976[3]** | | | | |
| 13–16 | 57.6 | 6.2 | 35.6 | 0.6 |
| 17 or more | 24.7 | 9.1 | 65.8 | 0.4 |
| **Private sector, 1976** | | | | |
| 13–16 | 90.3 | 0.3 | 9.2 | 0.2 |
| 17 or more | 46.2 | 1.2 | 52.4 | 0.2 |
| **Sweden, 1975–77[4]** | | | | |
| 13–16 | 18.2 | 9.2 | 72.6 | na |
| 17 or more | 2.1 | 27.2 | 70.7 | na |
| **United States, 1970–71[5]** | | | | |
| 13–16 | 39.4 | 7.9 | 51.4 | 1.3 |
| 17 or more | 0.0 | 4.4 | 94.5 | 1.1 |
| **United States, 1977[6]** | | | | |
| 13–16 | 66.7 | 0.9 | 32.1 | 0.3 |
| 17 or more | 10.0 | 0.8 | 88.5 | 0.7 |

1 Reported as suction or surgical curettage. Includes dilatation and evacuation (D & E) at 13 or more weeks of gestation.
2 Residents and nonresidents.
3 National Health Service hospitals.
4 Hysterotomy or hysterectomy refers to cases reported as 'other one-step methods' and medical induction to those reported as 'two-step methods.'
5 Data from the Joint Program for the Study of Abortion. Medical induction refers only to intra-amniotic instillation of hypertonic saline solution. The '0.0' entry at 17 weeks or more under dilatation and evacuation is an artifact since a few cases so reported were coded as of unknown gestation.
6 Based on reports from 28 states. Medical inductions include saline and prostaglandin and 90% of 'other procedures.' Abortions at 16 weeks subtracted from 16 weeks and over and added to 13–15 weeks by formula.

14% in 1977 in Canada, compared with 37% in the United States in 1970–71 and 55% in 1977.

Medical induction includes the intra- and extra-amniotic instillation of prostaglandin, hypertonic saline, and urea. In general, these procedures are used more often in the later than in the earlier part of the middle trimester; the exception is Sweden where extra-amniotic instillation is more widely practiced than in the other three countries. The use of medical induction has increased in England and Wales at the expense of hysterotomy; in the United States D&E is replacing some medical induction procedures.

As shown in Table 7, the ranking of prostaglandin, saline, and urea within the category of medical induction is quite different in different settings. Prostaglandin is the clear favorite in Britain's NHS-hospitals, while hypertonic saline predominates in Canada and especially in the United States. The private sector in England and Wales uses all three methods, with about equal frequency.

No national statistics on methods of abortion are collected in Japan. According to Professor Manabe (personal communication, 1979) of the Kyoto University School of Medicine the laminaria-metreurynter (balloon) combination is currently the most frequently used method for midtrimester abortions and probably over 80% are performed by this procedure which is gradually replacing extra-amniotic instillation of ethacridine lactate (Rivanol). The use of prostaglandins is increasing, but according to Muramatsu (personal communication, 1979), it is still mainly limited to academic institutions. Saline and urea are not used in Japan.

*Table 7.* Percent distribution of midtrimester medical inductions by method, within weeks of gestation: selected areas, 1977.

| Weeks of gestation | Prostaglandin | Saline | Urea |
|---|---|---|---|
| Canada | | | |
| 13–16 | 39.6 | 48.8 | 11.6 |
| 17 or more | 33.4 | 57.5 | 9.1 |
| England and Wales[1] | | | |
| 13–16 | 75.1 | 11.0 | 13.9 |
| 17 or more | 48.6 | 21.0 | 30.4 |
| NHS-hospitals | | | |
| 13–16 | 92.1 | 0.7 | 7.2 |
| 17 or more | 88.1 | 1.8 | 10.1 |
| Private sector | | | |
| 13–16 | 32.1 | 36.9 | 31.0 |
| 17 or more | 31.2 | 29.5 | 39.3 |
| United States[2] | | | |
| 13–16 | 25.1 | 66.3 | 8.6 |
| 17 or more | 29.1 | 64.2 | 6.7 |

[1] All 'other medical inductions' assumed to refer to urea.
[2] Ninety percent of 'other methods' assumed to refer to urea.

The different patterns exhibited in Tables 6 and 7 reflect, in the first instance, differences and changes in medical opinion and attitudes, generated in turn by the collective experience (or lack of it) of the profession, passed along in medical schools and teaching hospitals, modified occasionally by the communication of research findings through the network of professional channels of communication, and by the personal experience (or lack of it) of providers of abortion services Other and more subtle factors may be the organization of abortion services in the public and private sectors, the economic benefits or costs of specific procedures to providers and consumers, and the real or perceived risks of legal complications or administrative censure, to mention only a few

However, this is neither the place nor the time to document the specific circumstances and events shaping medical opinion and attitudes in each country at given periods Suffice it to say that in my opinion most midtrimester abortions reflect a personal or social failure, a failure on the part of the pregnant woman, her family, her doctor, the educational system, the medical system, the legal system, in fact, of society at large Any action or inaction or deliberate policy tending to delay the decision to seek abortion or to implement that decision increases the risks to life and health associated with the procedure

REFERENCES

1 Canada Statistics Canada *Therapeutic Abortions 1977* Also earlier volumes
2 Cates W Jr and Tietze C Standardized mortality rates associated with legal abortion United States, 1972 1975 *Fam Plann Perspect* 10 109–112, 1978
3 Czechoslovakia Institute for Health Statistics *Zdravotnicka Statistika CSSR Potraty 1977* Also earlier volumes
4 Forrest JD, et al Abortion in the United States, 1976–1977 *Fam Plann Perspect* 10 271–279, 1978
5 Hong SB and Tietze C Survey of abortion providers in Seoul, Korea *Stud Fam Plann* 10 161–163, 1979
6 Hungary Central Statistical Office *A Vetelesek Adatai 1974–1975* Also earlier volumes
7 Hungary Central Statistical Office *Terhessegmegszakitasok es Spontan Vetelesek Adatai 1976–1977*
8 India National Institute of Family Planning *Director s Report 1975–76*
9 Japan Ministry of Health and Welfare *Statistics of Eugenic Protection Showa 52* Also earlier volumes
10 Muramatsu M An analysis of factors in fertility control in Japan – an updated and revised version *Bull Inst Publ Health* 22 228–236, 1973
11 Pakter J, et al Legal abortion A half decade of experience *Fam Plann Perspect* 7 248–255, 1975, supplemented by unpublished data for 1975–77
12 Rao NB and Kanbagi R Legal abortion in an Indian State *Stud Fam Plann* 8 311–315, 1977, supplemented by unpublished data
13 Sweden National Board of Health and Welfare Aborter 1977 *Statistiska meddelanden,* HS 1979 5 Also earlier volumes and unpublished data for 1968 72

14 Tietze C and Lewit S Joint Program for the Study of Abortion (JPSA) Early medical complications of legal abortion *Stud Fam Plann* 3 97–122, 1972

15 Tietze C *Induced Abortion 1979* The Population Council, New York

16 United Kingdom Office of Population Censuses and Surveys *The Registrar General's Statistical Review of England and Wales Supplement on Abortion 1973* Also earlier volumes

17 United Kingdom Office of Population Censuses and Surveys *Abortion Statistics Legal abortions carried out under the 1967 Abortion Act in England and Wales, 1976* Also volumes for 1974 and 1975

18 United Kingdom Scottish Home and Health Department Abortion statistics *Health Bulletin* 35 282–295, 1977 Also earlier issues

19 United States Center for Disease Control *Abortion Surveillance 1977* Also earlier volumes

## 2. SECOND-TRIMESTER ABORTION AS A SOCIAL PROBLEM: DELAY IN ABORTION SEEKING BEHAVIOUR AND ITS CAUSES

### E. KETTING

Induced abortion after the 12th or 13th week of pregnancy has been an important subject of discussion for several years now. It is considered to be a problem in several respects. First, there is the controversy about the *moral acceptability* of induced abortion in general, which becomes more profound as the duration of pregnancy increases. Second, the *psychological problems* of pregnancy termination in the second trimester are often thought to be graver than during earlier stages of pregnancy. And third, the risk of *medical complications*, in general, increases with the duration of pregnancy although other factors, such as methods used and the level of experience of the physician, are also of crucial importance with respect to this risk.

The goal of scientific research, as in this field, should not be limited to the presentation of data but should be to supply these data with some meaning. With respect to this problem, it means that one of the major tasks of the social scientist is to find out why some women tend to delay in seeking abortion. The ultimate goal should be to prevent such delay as much as possible. In the same way that research among abortion patients in general should be directed toward finding out why unplanned pregnancies may not be prevented by means of contraception, research into the problem of second trimester abortion should be directed towards finding means to prevent delay.

Sociological research in this field has been concentrated upon two questions: 1) Which groups of patients show an increased risk in receiving treatment during a later stage of pregnancy? and 2) What are the reasons for this delay? I will try to answer these questions primarily with respect to the situation in Holland.

Due to legal barriers or a general lack of adequate facilities in their countries of residence, every year many women from abroad come to the Netherlands to have an abortion in one of the Dutch clinics. According to data from Stimezo* collected from practically all Dutch clinics in 1979, 32 000 German women, 7 500 Belgian women and 1 900 women from other countries (the majority from France) were treated here. Furthermore, 13 200 Dutch residents underwent an abortion in a clinic. An additional number of approxi-

---

* Stimezo-Nederland (National Abortion Federation of the Netherlands) is a non-profit organization of abortion clinics which aims at the improvement of public education in the field of family planning and of the quality of abortion services

*M J N C Keirse et al (eds ), Second Trimester Pregnancy Termination All rights reserved*
*Copyright © 1982 Martinus Nijhoff Publishers, The Hague/Boston/London*

mately 3 500 women were treated in a general or an academic hospital [1, 2].

The median duration of pregnancy was lowest among Dutch residents: 7.8 weeks; among German women it was 8.3 weeks, among Belgian women 8.4 weeks and among women from other countries 9.1 weeks. Table 1 shows that Dutch residents generally have an abortion at an earlier stage of pregnancy than foreign women. Twenty-three percent of the Dutch residents receive treatment in a hospital; unfortunately, adequate national statistics are not available for this group [2]. Thus, they are not included in this table. However, there are no indications that second trimester procedures are more frequent in hospitals than in clinics, although this is true for some individual, in particular academic, hospitals. The number of midtrimester abortions per 100 abortions among Dutch residents is rather low. Only in Sweden, Japan and some Eastern European countries have lower figures been reported [3]. However, as the incidence of abortion in general is extremely low in the Dutch population (5.6 per 1000 women aged 15–44 in 1979), the incidence of second trimester pregnancy termination is also very low, between 0.4 and 0.5 per 1000 women aged 15–44.

Probably the following three factors contribute to this low incidence:
1. The Dutch system of referral by the family doctor gives patients a quick access to a clinic. They do not have to search by themselves for a facility where the abortion can be performed.
2. In the clinics there are no unnecessary procedural or institutional barriers that could cause extra waiting time.
3. The clinics are evenly distributed over the country. Most family doctors know the clinic in their region and patients do not have to travel far [4].

For foreign patients the situation is quite different, which largely explains the fact that they tend to find help later in pregnancy. Although many foreign patients are directly referred to a Dutch clinic by their own physician, others have to find their way to a clinic without help from the medical profession, which often causes delay. Futhermore, many women can find help in their country of residence during the first trimester of pregnancy, but are forced to

Table 1. Percent distribution of abortions by weeks of gestation since last menstrual period and by country of residence: The Netherlands, 1979 and United States, 1976.

| | 8 weeks or less | 9–10 weeks | 11–12 weeks | 13–16 weeks | 17–20 weeks | 21 weeks or more |
|---|---|---|---|---|---|---|
| The Netherlands | 66.4 | 17.6 | 7.5 | 6.4 | 1.5 | 0.4 |
| West Germany | 53.3 | 24.0 | 11.1 | 8.6 | 2.6 | 0.4 |
| Belgium | 55.6 | 23.3 | 8.7 | 9.2 | 2.8 | 0.4 |
| Other countries | 41.9 | 22.5 | 11.0 | 16.1 | 7.0 | 1.5 |
| United States | 47.0 | 28.0 | 14.4 | 5.8 | 3.8 | 0.9 |

Source: Stimezo-Nederland (1980).

travel abroad if they have passed this period, for whatever reason. As Table 1 indicates, the outcome of these circumstances is that only 8.3% of the Dutch patients were second trimester cases, whereas among German, Belgian, and patients from other countries these percentages were 11.6, 12.4 and 24.6 respectively.

Data on Dutch patients who show an increased risk in delay are remarkably similar to those found in other areas. Everywhere an inverse relationship has been found between age of the patients and the risk in delay. As Table 2 shows, data on Dutch patients confirm this finding. Delay is a problem typical for adolescent girls. A further analysis with respect to age shows that the risk in delay increases up to the age of 16 and thereafter gradually decreases (not shown). It is not surprising that the risk in delay also correlates with marital status. This can be expected because of the age-distribution of second trimester cases (Table 3). Of course, age and marital status largely coincide. However, it is important to note that those who were once married (divorcées or widows) also tend to delay, although they are concentrated in the age group of women over thirty. A very important variable in this respect turns out to be the domestic circumstances of the woman. Table 4 shows that the risk of delay among those girls still living with their parents is, at almost 15%, nearly three times higher than among those

Table 2. Percentage of abortions on Dutch residents performed in the second trimester of pregnancy by age: 1979 (n = 13 206).

| Age | % |
| --- | --- |
| 14 years or less | 16.3 |
| 15–19 years | 14.5 |
| 20–24 years | 9.9 |
| 25–29 years | 7.3 |
| 30–34 years | 5.0 |
| 35–39 years | 5.0 |
| 40–44 years | 5.2 |
| 45 years or more | 7.0 |

Source: Stimezo-Nederland (1980)

Table 3. Percentage of abortions on Dutch residents performed in the second trimester of pregnancy by marital status: 1979 (n = 13 206).

| Marital status | % |
| --- | --- |
| Never married | 11.0 |
| Widowed | 10.9 |
| Divorced | 8.3 |
| Currently married | 5.6 |

Source: Stimezo-Nederland (1980)

*Table 4.* Percentage of abortions on Dutch residents performed in the second trimester of pregnancy according to domestic circumstances of the woman: 1979 (n = 13 206).

| Domestic circumstances | % |
|---|---|
| Living with parents | 14.8 |
| Living alone | 9.7 |
| Living alone with children | 8.6 |
| Living with partner and possible children | 5.3 |
| Other domestic circumstances | 13.9 |

Source: Stimezo-Nederland (1980)

women living with a partner, married or not. The risk of delay among women living alone lies between these two extremes. Research in different countries has also shown a relationship between prior pregnancy and incidence of late abortion. Since the number of prior pregnancies is of course strongly affected by the age of women, which in itself relates to the risk in delay, analysis at this point has been limited to the age group of women 20 or more years old. Within that age group it turns out that there is only a very weak relationship with prior experience of induced abortion. The number of living children, however, is a very discriminating variable, as is shown in Table 5. The relationship is U-shaped; women with two living children show a remarkably low risk in delay, while women without or with many children are quite often treated during the second trimester.

Finally, two other variables should be mentioned. Tietze and Lewitt [5], Bracken and Swigar [6], and Kerenyi et al. [7] have demonstrated that ethnic minorities show an increased risk in delay. The same holds for ethnic and cultural minorities in the Netherlands although the difference between them and the rest of the Dutch patients has decreased during recent years. Research in Britain and the United States has further shown that women from lower socio-economic classes and with a low level of education tend to delay in seeking an abortion [6, 8]. Schnabel [9] has demonstrated that the same applies to Dutch abortion patients.

Summarizing the data mentioned we can conclude that women most likely

*Table 5.* Percentage of abortions on Dutch residents performed in the second trimester of pregnancy by number of living children for women aged 20 years or more: 1979 (n = 10 893).

| Number of living children | % |
|---|---|
| 0 | 9.0 |
| 1 | 7.4 |
| 2 | 4.3 |
| 3 or more | 7.5 |

Source: Stimezo-Nederland (1980)

to delay abortion show the following characteristics:

1. Extremely young or over forty years old,
2. Unmarried or previously married,
3. Not living with a partner and especially those living with their parents,
4. Having no children or many children, and
5. Of low educational level and socio-economic class.

It should be remarked that these characteristics share a common denominator; they represent circumstances that are known to contribute to the unacceptability of pregnancy and parenthood. In my opinion this also points to the core of the moral problem concerning second trimester pregnancy termination: the general tendency is that *the later a woman applies for an abortion the more she is in need of it.*

Of course these socio-economic and demographic variables associated with delay do not explain the phenomenon. They only indicate where the problem is concentrated and more or less suggest what reasons could possibly be involved. Some research has been done in this field too. These reasons for delay can best be understood and systematically dealt with by focusing on the process of decision-making. Within this process at least three phases can be distinguished. They are: 1) recognition of pregnancy, 2) decision in favor of or against abortion, and 3) finding a facility where the abortion can be performed. Table 6 summarizes the main findings of five studies that included the question on reasons for delay. Three of them were American [7, 11, 12] and two were Dutch [10, 13]. During the first phase – recognition of pregnancy – denial of pregnancy and irregular menstruation are the most common reasons for delay. Unfamiliarity with pregnancy and incorrect diagnosis have also been found to be major reasons. Use of highly effective contraception as a

*Table 6* Major stated reasons (minimal and maximum percentages found) for delay in seeking abortion in five different studies (7, 10, 11, 12, 13)

| | min % | | max % |
|---|---|---|---|
| *First phase  recognition of pregnancy* | | | |
| denial of pregnancy (caused by extreme fear) | 7 5 | – | 22 5 |
| irregular menses (including supposed menopause) | 9 | – | 21 |
| Unfamiliar with the possibility of pregnancy | 8 | – | 14 |
| incorrect diagnosis of pregnancy | | 7 | |
| use of highly effective contraception | | 8 | |
| *Second phase  decision making* | | | |
| ambivalence, procrastination, etc | 14 | – | 27 |
| fear (to inform parents) | 7 5 | – | 20 |
| sudden change of circumstances | 2 | – | 12 |
| (foetal defects) | | | |
| *Third phase  finding an abortion facility* | | | |
| general lack of information | 4 5 | – | 9 |
| physician delay in referral | 6 | – | 16 |
| financial problems | 3 | – | 12 5 |
| (legal barriers or legally imposed waiting periods) | | | |

reason has only been found by Van de Bergh [10]. I will return to this problem below because it deserves some elaboration.

To a certain extent the reasons mentioned here explain why some of the aforementioned categories of patients tend to delay more than others. For instance, unfamiliarity with pregnancy and denial of this possibility is more likely to occur among nulliparous, young and sexually inexperienced patients than among others.

The same thing holds for reasons that may explain delay during the second phase. There, ambivalence is the reason most frequently stated. It is not difficult to imagine that it is easier to resolve such ambivalence for women who have a partner with whom they can discuss the problem than for those women who have to decide without adequate support. Hence, women living without a partner are generally more likely to have severe difficulties during the process of decision-making. Fear of informing their parents again explains why young girls constitute a high-risk group for delay. This fear can result in a kind of denial of pregnancy that is sometimes quite incredible. Finally, a woman is sometimes confronted with an abrupt change in her personal situation, such as the death of her partner, which can make a desired pregnancy suddenly highly unwanted.

During the third phase, lack of information about the possibilities of having a pregnancy terminated, delay in referral, sometimes deliberately, to a clinic or hospital and lack of financial means have been found to be major reasons. In Table 6 two other possibilities are added in parentheses. First, there is the possibility of second trimester pregnancy termination after pre-natal diagnosis of the fetus. Second, legal barriers may cause delay. In Dutch clinics this is seen every day. Foreign women often find their way to a Dutch clinic after having applied unsuccesfully for an abortion in their country of residence. Furthermore, legally imposed waiting periods — e.g. a week in France and five days in a recent Dutch abortion act — can cause delay. With respect to this problem, WHO has drawn the following conclusion: 'For maximal safety and efficiency, services should be available in such a way as to facilitate legal induction early in pregnancy by skilled operators. The greater the number of barriers to achieving this ideal, the greater the potential hazard to the health of the woman' [14].

One additional comment has to be made about Table 6. This table summarizes findings in the United States and in the Netherlands. However, there are some important differences between the two countries. First, the reasons found to explain delay during the third phase of abortion-seeking are much more frequent in the United States. Second, use of highly efficient contraception as a reason for delay has only been mentioned in one of the Dutch studies, which is probably not by accident. Contraceptive use in the Netherlands is far more efficient than in the United States. As a consequence the abortion rate is considerably lower; approximately five times as low. But this also means that a relatively large share of the abortion patients in the Netherlands have become pregnant in spite of the use of effective contraception. In 1979 about 24% of all Dutch patients claimed that a method failure of effective contraception (pill or IUD) or relatively effective contraception (condom or diaphragm) had been the cause of the unwanted pregnancy. On the other hand 26.3% had not used any kind of contraception. The rest, about half the number of patients, had used ineffective means of contraception or reported patient failures with more effective contraceptives. The relationship between contraceptive use and delay in seeking an abortion has been studied by Oppel et al. [15], who found a higher frequency of contraceptive use among early abortion patients. Treffers et al. [13] came to a similar finding for Dutch patients. Table 7 confirms this general tendency. The risk in delay decreases as contraceptive use improves. Among those not using contraception, 10% were treated in the second trimester of pregnancy. In the patient-failure group this was 8% and in the method-failure group only 4%. However, if we look at the reliability of the methods used, we arrive at the opposite conclusion: women who use reliable methods show a higher risk in delay than those who use unreliable methods. Particularly in cases of method failure, there is a great difference between groups. These data can be regarded as a confirmation of the hypothesis that the use of highly effective contraception may make a woman think that the possibility of pregnancy is out of the question. Therefore, it is important that women are given adequate information on this point.

Finally, the conclusions that may be drawn from these data and investigations are essentially twofold:

1. Second trimester abortion facilities are indispensable from a social point of

*Table 7* Percent distribution of abortions on Dutch residents by weeks of gestation (since last menstrual period) and by contraceptive use prior to abortion for women aged 20 years or more (1979)

| Contraceptive use prior to abortion | 8 weeks or less | 9–12 weeks | 13–16 weeks | 17 weeks or more | Total % | No |
|---|---|---|---|---|---|---|
| No use | 63 | 27 | 7 | 3 | 100 | 1825 |
| Patient failure | 65 | 26 | 6 | 2 | 100 | 1032 |
| 1) unreliable method | 76 | 20 | 3 | 1 | 100 | 192 |
| 2) relatively reliable method | 80 | 15 | 3 | 1 | 100 | 267 |
| 3) reliable method | 55 | 33 | 8 | 3 | 100 | 573 |
| Method failure | 75 | 21 | 3 | 1 | 100 | 3681 |
| 1) unreliable method | 76 | 22 | 2 | - | 100 | 2087 |
| 2) relatively reliable method | 77 | 19 | 3 | 1 | 100 | 1022 |
| 3) reliable method | 68 | 23 | 6 | 3 | 100 | 573 |
| Total | 70 | 24 | 5 | 2 | 100 | 6538 |

Source Stimezo-Nederland (1980)

view, because the second trimester cases are the ones that tend to be most in need of help the very young girls, the poor, the women who do not have a partner, the women with many children, etc

2 Incentives and government measures to prevent delay are badly needed and can be useful Such measures should be mainly directed toward the following goals

a the improvement of sexual, reproductive and contraceptive education

b the improvement of information on existing possibilities for pregnancy termination

c the increase in the motivation of professional health-workers not to delay their services unnecessarily in cases of unwanted pregnancy, and last but not least

d the establishment of provisions for abortion and related services Neither institutional nor legal barriers to second trimester pregnancy termination should exist, because international data show that the incidence of second trimester abortion is lowest in those countries where abortion in general is most easily available

REFERENCES

1 Ketting E and Schnabel P Induced abortion in the Netherlands a decade of experience *Stud Fam Plann* 11 385–394, 1980

2 Kolkman-Koelink B and Ketting E *Abortus provocatus in het ziekenhuis* NISSO, Zeist, 1980

3 Tietze C *Induced Abortion 1979* (3rd edn) The Population Council, New York, 1979

4 Ketting E *Late Abortus in Nederland* Stimezo Den Haag, 1979

5 Tietze C and Lewit S Joint program for the study of abortion (JPSA) early medical complications of legal abortion *Stud Fam Plann* 3 97–122, 1972

6 Bracken MB and Swigar ME Factors associated with delay in seeking induced abortions *Am J Obstet Gynecol* 113 301–309, 1972

7 Kerenyi TD, Glascock EL and Horowitz ML Reasons for delayed abortion results of four hundred interviews *Am J Obstet Gynecol* 117 299–311, 1973

8 Johnson FD and Vincent L Factors affecting gestational age at termination of pregnancy *Lancet* 1 717, 1973

9 Schnabel P *Abortus in Nederland* Stimezo, Den Haag, 1976

10 Van de Bergh AS *De Methode 'Finks en Alternatieve Technieken voor Therapeutische Zwangerschapsafbreking in het Tweede Trimester van de Graviditeit* Stimezo, Den Haag, 1977

11 Fielding WL, Sachtleben MR, Friedman LM and Friedman EA Comparison of women seeking early and late abortion *AM J Obstet Gynecol* 131 304–310, 1978

12 Mallory GB, Rubenstein LZ, Drosness DL, Kleiner GJ and Sidel VW Factors responsible for delay in obtaining interruption of pregnancy *Obstet Gynecol* 40 556–562, 1972

13 Treffers PE, Van de Berg GR, Jager-van Gelder PA and Van Oenen JJ Abortusverzoeken in het tweede trimester van de graviditeit *Ned Tijdschr Geneesk* 120 2255–2263, 1976

14 WHO Scientific Group *Induced Abortion* Technical Report Series 623, WHO Geneva 1978

15 Oppel W, Athanasiou R, Cushner I Sasaki T, Unger T and Wolf S Contraceptive antecedents to early and late therapeutic abortions *Am J Publ Health* 62 824–827, 1972

# 3. LEGAL ASPECTS OF PREGNANCY TERMINATION IN EUROPE

PAUL SCHNABEL

## 1. INTRODUCTION

Discussing the legal aspects of pregnancy termination has become part of the historical and cultural heritage of this country. The discussion has been going on for about a century and still there seems to be no definite and satisfying solution to the problem of abortion on request or demand. The Dutch abortion laws date from 1886 and 1911, and since 1970 there have been no less than eight attempts to revise these old and completely obsolete laws. Unfortunately, up till now all attempts have failed, with the rather odd consequence that the Netherlands is now one of the last countries in western Europe waiting for a liberalization of its abortion laws, while at the same time maintaining an abortion policy that may be considered most liberal. In this country abortion on request is generally and easily available for residents as well as for non-residents in the first and in the second trimester of pregnancy.

Though this paradoxical situation may be typical for the Netherlands, there can be no doubt that the process of liberalizing the existing abortion laws has been a long and very difficult one in nearly all countries of western Europe. One of the main reasons for this is the very existence of these laws. If there had been no abortion laws at all, as was the case in most countries up to the end of the nineteenth century, we would not now witness such a harsh and aggressive discussion on liberalization and the moral acceptability of elective abortion. This point may need some clarification.

In the Netherlands every year more than 100 000 men and women choose voluntary sterilization. This figure outnumbers the number of abortions more than five times. Furthermore, sterilization is virtually irreversible, whereas abortion normally does not have any repercussions on reproductive capability. In spite of all these differences, which mean that sterilization has many more consequences than abortion, nobody discusses the legal aspects of sterilization, as there are no legal aspects to be discussed or, more correctly, there are no specific legal aspects to be discussed beyond the general laws regulating medical practice. A plea for the introduction of a law on sterilization is hardly ever heard. In contrast to this, the 17 000 abortions performed each year on Dutch women have constituted a major political issue for more than a decade. The reason for this is not only that abortion, more than sterilization, is an ethical problem – it certainly is considered to be so by many – but also that abortion has traditionally been subject to a prohibitive law and sterilization has not. It is easier to come to terms with a completely new situation that has never been regulated before, neither negatively nor positively, than to accept a major change in an existing law which in its original form expresses a deeply felt moral position even if it is by now the position of a minority. It must be added, however, that due to the influence of the growing medical profession in its struggle for a monopoly in the field of health care, restrictive abortion laws were introduced in most western countries at the end of the 19th century.

In no European country has the final step been made towards a complete decriminalization and depenalization of abortion. On the contrary, in most countries the old abortion laws, which mostly stated quite clearly that abortion was not allowed and that in case of breaking the law both woman and provider would be prosecuted, have been replaced by statutes regulating abortion and abortion procedures in detail. Generally speaking, these regulations are meant to make elective abortion anything but easy. In other words, the recently adopted abortion laws are mostly a mixture of political compromises, with little mutual coherence and in no way intended to improve the quality of the abortion services. Legalization of abortion is a way of making abortion difficult. Most modern abortion laws state in great detail where, when and on whom abortion may be performed. Abortion is one of the very few medical acts to be made subject to extramedical control as a normal procedure. Normally, medical acts are performed by the doctor in accordance with the rules of his profession and with the patient's consent.

COMPONENTS OF MODERN ABORTION LAWS

A most effective and efficient way to depenalize abortion would be simply to consider abortion as an integral part of normal medical practice, subject to the rules pertaining to this practice. Termination of pregnancy would then fall in the same range as e.g. the removal of an appendix, at least from a legal point of view. The moral aspects of pregnancy termination would then be an extralegal problem, to be solved by mutual arrangement between the doctor and his patient. Normally, the doctor needs the patient's consent to perform any operation that he considers to be necessary. In the case of pregnancy termination, the patient needs the doctor's consent to have the requested operation done. This certainly makes an important difference. But it remains to be seen if this difference makes the interference of the legislator really inevitable.

In all countries where abortion has become legalized in one way or another, the legislator has in fact considerably increased his influence on the abortion practice. The new abortion laws may specify the following points:

1. *The formal procedures* to be followed in the process of decision-making. The procedures may point out who is going to decide on the abortion (the patient, the doctor, a special committee); whether it is necessary to secure a second opinion (as is the case in England and Wales); or whether there will be a waiting period between the decision and the operation itself.

2. *The grounds for termination.* These consist of the well-known *indications* for abortion, mostly divided into medical, eugenic, juridical, psychiatric, economic, psychosocial and social indications. A medical indication — abortion to preserve the life or physical health of the mother — is always considered to be a 'hard' indication, which means that an abortion is undisputably necessary. A social indication, however, is considered to be 'soft'; the criteria for the evaluation of the social condition of the patient are vague and arbitrary.

In eastern Europe and Scandinavia we also find another ground for termination: age of the woman and number of children. In these cases, abortion on request is available if the woman has reached a certain age or already has a family of above average size. For instance, in Czechoslovakia abortion is legal if the woman is over 40, if she is a widow or if she has at least three children. In Finland abortion is legal if the woman is under 17 or over 40, or if she already has four children. These are mere *conditions* instead of indications.

In some cases, the legislator has decided not to specify grounds for termination at all. In fact, quite a few of the more recent abortion laws explicitly or implicitly accept *abortion on request,* but only up to a certain duration of pregnancy. After 10–13 weeks pregnancy abortion is only legal if performed under rather strict indications.

3. *The eligibility for an abortion licence.* Some laws state the criteria that have to be met by the doctor, the institution or the hospital in order to get permission to perform abortions, to counsel patients who want to have an abortion, or to procure referral letters. These criteria can be formal (e.g. the institution must be a non-profit one; the medical director must be a gynaecologist; abortion may not constitute more than a certain percentage of all the operations performed; abortion may only be performed in a general hospital) or material, which means that the institution must have certain equipment or facilities at its disposal (e.g. a fully equipped operating theatre, a defibrillator, facilities for general anaesthesia).

4. *The services to be rendered.* Sometimes the legislator requires in detail the provision of some special services for the patient. This may consist of an obligation to inform the patient about possibilities other than termination of the pregnancy. It may also be that the legislator requires a clinical setting for the operation or makes counseling on matters of family planning obligatory.

5. *The notification and inspection.* For statistical reasons, but certainly also for reasons of control and inspection, most new abortion laws require notification of the abortions performed to the Ministry of Health or another official agency. In some cases, abortionists and abortion clinics are subject to stricter control by the State Inspection of Health than other providers of health care.

6. *The penalties and sanctions.* It is interesting to note that with most modern abortion laws the woman concerned is no longer subject to prosecution. With respect to the abortion clinics and the doctors concerned, the modern laws are considerably less lenient. In many cases, they must be prepared to pay high fines for comparatively light administrative errors. A clinic may even lose its licence, and in cases of serious medical error — not necessarily malpractice – the doctor may even risk a long sentence.

Generally speaking, the new abortion laws convey an attitude of distrust towards the doctors who perform abortions and their women-patients. Legalization of pregnancy termination without any restriction is feared to give way to the use of abortion as contraceptive practice par excellence and to ruthless exploitation by the medical profession of the need for abortion. This attitude of apparent distrust has materialized in a whole catalogue of regulations and sanctions, which emphasizes the exceptionality of abortion. Abortion is the 'last' and the 'least' solution to unwanted pregnancy.

ABORTION LAWS IN EUROPE AND THE USA

There is a widespread belief that the liberalized abortion laws constitute a definite break in an old and firmly established tradition of antiabortion legislation. This is only partly true. In many countries the traditional abortion laws are remnants of late 19th century efforts to improve public and personal moral sense by laws. The validity of these efforts has always been questioned and the enactment of restrictive abortion laws has always been followed by attempts to decriminalize abortion as well as by pleas for the provision of adequate contraception. At the end of the 19th century most western countries had introduced abortion laws into their Penal Codes and in the first half of the 20th century these laws became even more strict. This was not the case in the Nordic and eastern European countries, as we will see below.

In western Europe, the United Kingdom (excluding Northern Ireland) was the first country to renew its abortion legislation [2]. In 1967 a new abortion law was enacted authorizing abortion on specified but not very clear grounds. The Abortion Act states the following:

'... a person shall not be guilty of an offence under the law relating to abortion when a pregnancy is terminated ... if two registered medical practitioners are of the opinion, formed in good faith

a) that the continuance of the pregnancy would involve risk to the life of the pregnant woman or of injury to the physical or mental health of the pregnant woman or any existing children of her family, greater than if the pregnancy were terminated; or

b) that there is a substantial risk that if the child were born it would suffer from such physical or mental abnormalities as to be seriously handicapped'.

The passus 'greater than if the pregnancy were terminated' in a peculiar way became of supreme importance, as the development of new abortion techniques, especially the suction method, brought about the fact that continuance of any pregnancy would involve more risks to the health of the woman than termination would. As most of the new techniqes were only developed after 1967, the Abortion Act and its subsequent statutory instruments and regulations were soon surpassed by the innovations. The Abortion Act at that time necessarily supposes abortion to be an operation in a clinical setting, a hospital. Pregnancy termination on an outpatient basis could not come into operation in Britain and this is still so, although the suction method is in regular use. This is but one problem of the positive legalization of abortion: it does not account for medical innovation and so may hamper the introduction of better and cheaper ways of terminating a pregnancy.

Great Britain set the trend, but certainly not the pace. After 1967 abortion became a political issue in all other countries of western Europe, and a very important one as it became clear that many women from the continent went to Britain to obtain an abortion (up to nearly 60 000 in 1973 and 31 000 in 1977 [3]. The liberalization of abortion took many years in most countries and,

Table 1 Abortion legislation in Europe and the USA (1980)

| 1 | Abortion is not permitted or only permitted on medical grounds | Ireland, Albania, Spain, Portugal Belgium, Switzerland, the Netherlands |
|---|---|---|
| 2 | Abortion is permitted on other than medical grounds (eugenic, juridical, social, psychological, economical) or on specified conditions (age, parity, marital status) | *Strict* Greece, Romania, Bulgaria, Turkey<br>*Liberal* Poland, Czechoslovakia, Iceland, German Federal Republic, Hungary, Finland, Great Britain |
| 3 | Abortion is permitted on request (no grounds specified) | Austria, Denmark, Norway, Sweden, France, Yugoslavia, USSR, German Democratic Republic, Luxemburg, USA |

surprisingly, it was Austria that in 1975, first, followed the British example. Abortion on request is now legal in Austria during the first trimester of pregnancy. In recent years new abortion laws have been enacted in France (1975, 1979), the Federal Republic of Germany (1976), Italy (1978) and Luxemburg (1979).

In 1980, the only countries in *western Europe* still having (very) restrictive abortion laws prohibiting abortion under practically all circumstances (with the possible exception of abortion on strictly medical grounds) are Ireland, Albania, Spain, Portugal, Belgium, Switzerland and the Netherlands. With the exception of Ireland and Albania, abortion in all these countries is a heavily discussed and controversial subject. The influence of the Roman Catholic Church on the political constellation in most of these countries (including the Netherlands, where 40% of the population belongs to the Roman Catholic Church) especially impedes the liberalization of abortion statutes. In Switzerland, there is considerable differentiation in interpretation of the law between the cantons.

By contrast, in the *Nordic* countries (Denmark, Norway, Sweden, Finland and Iceland) definite steps toward a liberalization of abortion were already taken before World War II and since then there has been a gradual development toward abortion on request. Some countries, however, do not allow abortion in the second trimester simply on the request of the patient alone. The abortion facilities in these countries are not normally open to women from abroad.

If we turn to the *socialist* countries of eastern Europe, the scenery changes dramatically. In 1955, abortion was liberalized in the USSR for the second time since the Revolution in 1917 (in the Stalinist period a more restrictive abortion policy was adopted). The new liberal policy was taken over by practically all other socialist countries, with the exception of the German Democratic Republic. In recent years however, Hungary, Romania, Bulgaria and Czechoslavakia quite suddenly reversed their liberal attitudes toward abortion and as a consequence of their concern about the ever-declining birthrates between 1966 and 1973, they adopted new and much more restrictive laws. In the German Democratic Republic however, abortion is now permitted on request in the first trimester of pregnancy. Only Yugoslavia and Poland have not witnessed changes in their abortion laws in the last ten years.

In the *socialist* countries abortion laws are clearly an instrument of population policy. Restrictive measures greatly affect the life of the people in these countries, as effective contraception is still hard to come by. For many women and couples in the socialist countries, abortion is the only available method of family planning.

The legal situation in the *United States of America* is rather difficult to grasp. In the majority (about 30) of the states abortion is only permitted to save the life of the mother. Some states have very liberal laws (California, New York) and in 1973 the Supreme Court ruled that, while there is no absolute constitutional right to abortion, abortion in the first trimester of pregnancy is to be decided on by the woman (and the doctor) alone. The state has no right to curtail her freedom on this point; however, in the second trimester of pregnancy the state may regulate abortion. While the state does not have the right to prohibit abortion in the first trimester of pregnancy, it has no obligation whatsoever to provide the necessary services, nor to refund the cost of an abortion.

TIME LIMITS FOR ABORTION

Table 2 gives an overview of the great differences in time limits set to abortion in various countries. The already complex situation is further complicated by the fact that the actual policy in most countries tends to keep a safe distance from the time limits. Furthermore, as there is no international uniform standard for assessing the period of gestation, there is considerable variety within and between countries in the interpretation of 'period of gestation'. In some countries it is normal practice to consider the number of weeks since the onset of the last menstrual period as the duration of the pregnancy (the amenorrhea model), in other countries the actual duration of the pregnancy (as assessed after the operation) is the criterion (the gestation model). The difference between the two models can be considerable. Generally speaking the duration of the pregnancy according to the amenorrhea model is a safeguard against involuntary crossing of the time limit.

*Table 2.* Abortion legislation and duration of pregnancy.

| | |
|---|---|
| 8 weeks: | Iceland |
| 10 weeks: | France, Bulgaria |
| 12 weeks: | Denmark, Norway (I), Finland, Austria, F.R. Germany (I), Romania, Yugoslavia, Hungary, Poland, USSR |
| 13 weeks: | Italy |
| 18 weeks: | Sweden, Norway (II) |
| 22 weeks: | F.R. Germany (II) |

From Table 2, it is easy to infer that there are three different policies:
a) no time limit at all, abortion being permitted prior to the viability of the foetus (Great Britain, USA, the Netherlands);
b) a time limit for abortion on request or on 'soft' indications (in the first trimester of pregnancy) and a time limit for strictly medical abortion in the second trimester of pregnancy: Federal Republic of Germany, Norway;

c) a limit for abortion on request or on 'soft' indications (in the first trimester of pregnancy), but no specified upper time limit for strictly medical abortion: all other countries.

It may be concluded from Table 2 that while there is considerable variation between countries in time limits for abortion, there is a strong tendency to liberalize abortion in the first trimester of pregnancy. In most countries abortion in the second trimester of pregnancy is only allowed on medical or eugenic grounds (continuation of pregnancy as a direct threat to the life of the mother or as a severe threat to the woman's physical and mental health; genetic or other impairment of the foetus, or risk of impairment). Some countries permit abortion in the second trimester, if the pregnancy is to be considered as a sequel of rape or incest. Only in Sweden, Great Btitain, the Netherlands and the USA is there a more liberal attitude towards abortion in the second trimester. This liberality, though, is not always in complete agreement with the apparent opinion of the legislator. For all practical purposes however, one may say that in these four countries abortion in the second trimester is certainly more than a mere theoretical possibility. The abortion services in Great Britain and the Netherlands are in fact the last resorts for women from all over Europe, desperately in need of an abortion in the second trimester of pregnancy.

ABORTION LAWS AND ABORTION POLICIES

Abortion laws do not always mirror the actual abortion situation. In most countries with very restrictive laws criminal abortion is widespread, while in some countries, such as the Netherlands and, in a very subtle way, Belgium, a restrictive law is frustrated by a liberal policy. On the other hand, many countries with a liberal law do not succeed or do not want to succeed in providing the necessary facilities. Abortion on request is now easily available in Austria, Skandinavia, Great Britain, the Netherlands, the USA and some socialist countries. Abortion on request is available, but not always easily obtainable in France, the Federal Republic of Germany, Italy and Luxemburg. It is still difficult to obtain abortion on request in Belgium, and very difficult or impossible in countries such as Spain, Portugal and Ireland.

The situation in the Netherlands needs some clarification [4]. The Dutch Penal Code of 1886 and 1911 forbids abortion explicitly. In accordance with the prevailing philosophy of law no exception has been made in the law to allow abortion on strictly medical grounds, as it is taken for granted that abortion on medical grounds may always be performed. In such cases there is an extralegal excuse, if the doctor can make a plausible case that he has acted in accordance with the rules of his profession. As within the medical profession the concept 'medical' in general has gradually lost its strictly physiological meaning, this holds for abortion as well So, nowadays a doctor is not only safeguarded by the law if he performs an abortion to save the mother's life, but also if he performs an abortion on any other ground considered acceptable by the medical profession in general This means in practice that abortion is 'legal' if performed by a doctor with the patient's consent The political discussion now is between liberals who want to make legitimate and regulate the present situation, and conservatives, who want to re-establish the abortion laws in their original and stricter interpretation It does seem however, that many conservatives are now slowly moving towards a more liberal attitude and the main problem will be exactly how far a new law will make the present situation legitimate Table 3 presents an overview of the bills that have been presented to the Dutch parliament in the last decade

Liberalization of abortion laws and policies is still an ongoing process in many countries Although it is expected that within a few years abortion will become generally available in nearly all European countries, this certainly does not imply that restrictive tendencies will lose their influence On the contrary, in many countries with a liberal practice or a new abortion act, strong efforts are made to curb abortion and to amend the abortion statutes in a more conservative way In the USA (no abortion refunding through Medicaid) and in F R Germany (intervention of the Constitutional Court) these attempts have been quite successful An attempt to bring in a time limit of 24 weeks in the British Abortion Act did not succeed In France the abortion law of 1975 nearly perished in a political conflict between left and right In the Netherlands it turned out to be politically difficult to adapt an obsolete abortion law to the practice of liberal abortion that had developed

Abortion is a problem with so many important ethical, political, medical and social aspects that it is very unlikely ever to find a political solution acceptable to society as a whole Quite understandably, this holds even more for the specific case of abortion in the second trimester

REFERENCES

1 Ketting E *Van Misdrijf tot Hulpverlening – Een Analyse van de Maatschappelijke Betekenis van Abortus Provocatus in Nederland* Samsom, Alphen a d Rijn, 1978
2 Report of the Committee on the Working of the Abortion Act (Lange Committee), I, 190–224 HMSO, London, 1974
3 Tietze C *Induced Abortion 1979* Population Council, New York, 1979
4 Ketting E and Schnabel P Induced abortion in the Netherlands a decade of experience *Stud Fam Plann*, 11 (1980) 12, 385–394

*Table 3* Bills for a new Abortion Act, the Netherlands, 1970–1980

| Bill proposed by | Year | Political background | Main issues | Fate (1981) |
|---|---|---|---|---|
| 1 Lambers/Roethof | 1970 | Members of Parliament (socialists) | Decriminalization of abortion | Merged in 5 |
| 2 Stuyt/Van Agt | 1972 | Government (Christian democrats & conservatives) | Medical indication (broad) second and third opinion | Withdrawn in 1975 |
| 3 Van Schaik/Van Leeuwen | 1975 | Members of Parliament (Christian democrats) | Medical indication (broad), abortion committee | Withdrawn in 1976 |
| 4 Veder-Smit/Geurtsen | 1975 | Members of Parliament (conservatives) | Abortion on request, abortion facilities strictly supervised by a national committee, abortion remains in the Penal Code | Merged in 5 |
| 5 Geurtsen/Lambers/Roethof/Veder-Smit | 1976 | Members of Parliament (conservatives & socialists) | Abortion on request, general supervision of the abortion facilities by a national committee | Passed in the House of Representatives, defeated in the Senate, 1976 |
| 6 Ginjaar/De Ruiter | 1979 | Government (Christian democrats & conservatives) | Abortion on request, five days after the request, special license for abortion clinics | Bill accepted 1981, to be enacted in 1982 |
| 7 Abma/Verbrugh | 1979 | Members of Parliament (conservative Protestants) | Abortion only on medical indication (very strictly interpreted) | Rejected 1980 |
| 8 Roethof/Wessel-Tuinstra | 1980 | Members of Parliament (socialists & liberals) | Abortion on request, some formal regulations for abortion facilities | Would have been discussed, if 6 had not been adopted |

# 4. A REVIEW OF ABORTION PRACTICES AND THEIR SAFETY

## PETER DIGGORY

Abortion has been reported throughout recorded history, and there is ar-
chaeological evidence for its use as long ago as the middle kingdom of Ancient
Egypt. Excavations at Pompeii have recovered a form of vaginal speculum
and instruments which are certainly very suitable for its performance. Unfortunately our knowledge as to the extent of abortion practice is very largely
anecdotal with nothing upon which to base even an informed guess as to
numbers until modern times. When cultural attitudes were permissive, and
legislation was largely non-existent, we gain from contemporary literature an
impression of fairly widespread abortion, often with some indications of the
techniques used. Classical scholars may recollect Ovid's lament that 'there are
few women nowadays who bear all the children they conceive'. Under regimes
which were culturally and legally repressive abortion undoubtedly continued,
but our knowledge is fragmentary and contemporary writers rarely referred
to it.

Anecdotally, potions have often been mentioned, and there is a tendency to
believe that the Ancient Egyptians, the Romans, and various tribal peoples
knew of effective drugs which could reliably procure abortion. In fact, there is
no evidence for such beliefs, and it is probably that if truly effective abortifacients had ever been discovered, their continued usage would have prevented the secrets of their constitution being lost. We have the same problem
in modern times in that various concoctions have been sold and eagerly
bought, as Cole and his colleagues dramatically showed in 1966 [1], but when
their constitution is considered it is clear that they are totally ineffective, and
that the recommendation they have received must have been due either to
coincidental miscarriage, or to the fact that the women who 'successfully'
took them were not in fact pregnant in the first place. In the late nineteenth
century the widespread use of lead salts, ergot preparations, quinine and
strong purgatives as abortifacients may have contributed to abortion, but in
individual cases failure of such medicaments must have greatly exceeded
success. Throughout the ages it would seem that effective abortion has primarily been instrumental, as it still is.

Recently Tongplaew Narkavonkit [2], described the technique of massage
abortion as practised in Thailand and claimed that 240 000 abortions are
performed there annually in this way. In western countries most of us have

seen women who have had successful abortions by a form of vigorous abdomino-uterine compression or massage, and probably such methods have been used since ancient times. Actual instrumentation involves such procedures as douching, introduction of instruments or foreign bodies into the uterine cavity, rupture of membranes, insertion of intra-uterine pastes or fluids, or the deliberate destruction of the foetus, either by somewhat indiscriminate injury, or by finding the umbilical cord and cutting it. All these techniques were in evidence in the U.K. twenty years ago, and are still much practised in various parts of the world. As an example, the traditional method of abortion in England at the turn of the century was the introduction of a crochet hook which was manoeuvred inside the uterus disrupting the embryo. This technique is still much used in the Howrah district of Calcutta. The preferred instrument is identical in all respects as crochet-work is one of the cottage industries of the city. In rural India abortion by the insertion of a fire-hardened straight twig is commonly practised.

The transcervical intrauterine injection of fluids is a fairly recent form of abortion since it requires a suitable form of syringe or water pump. The rubber 'enema syringe' was the commonly used instrument in Britain until very recently, and is probably still used occasionally today. I have seen examples of the same technique in Cairo and Italy and imagine that its use was widespread. The introduction of foreign bodies such as the rolled bark of trees is commonly used in India, and was a technique in Europe fifty years ago. One could go on recounting methods which were reputedly used here in the past, and are still in use today in various less developed parts of the world. It is obvious that within a small community those whose methods are the least likely to be infective or harmful rapidly gain credence, and that these safer techniques are then passed on over the generations, evolving rapidly as more suitable materials become locally available. We could describe the process as one of scientific development hampered by lack of adequate publicity, and we might then reflect that western medicine proceeded in the very same manner until very recently when abortion gained respectability and acceptance, and different techniques were reported and contrasted with proper scientific scrutiny, leading to the enormous improvement in abortion mortality and morbidity in the last decade.

Mohr [3] in his comprehensive and scholarly book 'Abortion in America' writes primarily about the social and political factors which caused American women to lose for the century from about 1870 to 1970 what had previously been widely regarded as their tacit right to abortion. His voluminous coverage of the social scene illustrates the development of advertised and obviously tolerated criminal abortion organisations, but even Mohr has been unable to quantify the incidence of such abortions. Very many attempts have been made to do so on demographic grounds, and the work of Beric [4] in Yugoslavia has shown how regional variations in birth rates are attributable primarily to the use of abortion, at first when it was illegal, and now officially approved. In 1966 Professor Rhodes [5] of St Thomas's Hospital, London estimated 100 000 criminal abortions in England and Wales, and suggested that the mortality might be as low as 50 women per year, this being at a time when childbirth in England carried a risk of 25 deaths per 100 000 deliveries. Rhodes felt that illegal abortion was not demonstrably more liable than childbirth to result in pelvic sepsis, and that in general the social cost of criminal abortion was not as high as passion might suggest.

Because reliable data were simply not available, and even in the 1960s the number of criminal abortions was still the subject of widely varying estimates, I shall presume to give you some data from my own experience. In 1958 I first came to Kingston Hospital, which is on the outskirts of London with a surrounding district of about 270 000 people, most of whom come to us for all their hospital needs, and all of whom would normally come if they needed to be admitted to hospital as an emergency. At that time not more than three or four therapeutic abortions were performed per year. Abortion was available by private doctors, but the ambiguity of the law led to high charges, and for poor, and even for lower middle-class women, the option was either to accept an unwanted pregnancy or to seek help illegally. Yet it was even then known that abortion was the commonest cause of the death of a pregnant woman, and that a previous criminal abortion was the commonest cause of female infertility.

In 1958 very little work had been done to determine how many illegal abortions were being performed. I failed then, as I have failed now, to find any reliable statistics preceding this data. Criminal abortion is a particularly difficult field of study. It is often absolutely impossible to establish whether a given woman is having a spontaneous or an induced abortion. I well remember one woman who, though gravely ill, maintained that her abortion was spontaneous right up to the time when she was given the last rites by her priest and yet, when the foetus was expelled and she began to recover, a rubber catheter came with it.

In 1965 I studied all our abortion admissions and personally interviewed every such woman, stressing that anything she told me would be completely confidential, and that neither the police nor relatives would be informed with out permission. During the year we had 1384 gynaecological admissions of which 397 were cases of abortion. The high quality of local family doctors meant that most spontaneous abortions were treated at home. 241 women actually admitted that their abortion was induced either by themselves or by someone else acting illegally. There were a few women who steadfastly refused to admit interference, but whose condition and progress made it certain that in fact the abortion had been criminally induced; I have already mentioned one of them. There is no doubt that more than 250 cases of criminal abortion were admitted by us in 1965.

Having seen so many criminal abortions and their complications, particularly the guilt and terror which usually accompanied them, I realised that desperate women always do obtain abortion of an unwanted pregnancy, and I felt that if such abortions were to be done then I could and should do them better than the criminal abortionist. Perhaps my early experience, before our law was liberalised, may be of interest in showing the techniques available and the complications which occurred.

Between mid-1964 and mid-1968 I carried out 1000 consecutive therapeutic abortions [6]. These were a selected group not reflecting national figures. My series included 18 doctors, 84 students, 29 teachers and 42 schoolgirls. Nevertheless, the social class distribution corresponded surprisingly well with the national figures, except for a loading in social class one. The age distribution was much as expected. The techniques used are interesting to review (Table 1). I tried vacuum aspiration but only with very primitive apparatus and inadequate suction, and abandoned it because three out of seven patients had to return to theatre for a curettage. I already regarded hypertonic saline as potentially unsafe and preferred utus paste introduced through the cervix. The technique involved passing a long fine-bore cannula and the paste came supplied in what looked like a large tube of toothpaste. Simple curettage was used in 77% of cases and hysterotomy in 16%. There were four serious complications, three definite perforations of the uterus, none requiring laparotomy, and one burst abdomen after hysterotomy (Table 2).

During the years 1964–68 I also noted details of various criminal abortion techniques which had been used by or upon those of my patients who were willing to discuss such details. I believe that there were probably about four criminal abortions successfully induced without complications necessitating hospital admission for every woman who came under my care. This was also

Table 1. 1000 consecutive abortions in 1964–1968, analysed by method of termination and by age.

| | ≤16 | 16–20 | 21–25 | 26–30 | 31–35 | 36–40 | 41–45 | ≥46 | Total |
|---|---|---|---|---|---|---|---|---|---|
| Vaginal termination | 22 | 190 | 259 | 115 | 92 | 63 | 28 | 1 | 770 |
| Hysterotomy | 3 | 20 | 11 | 9 | 0 | 1 | 0 | 1 | 45 |
| Hysterotomy and sterilisation | 0 | 0 | 4 | 14 | 38 | 38 | 18 | 2 | 114 |
| Utus paste | 4 | 22 | 19 | 7 | 6 | 1 | 0 | 0 | 59 |
| Intra-amniotic hypertonic saline | 1 | 0 | 2 | 1 | 1 | 0 | 0 | 0 | 5 |
| Suction curette | 0 | 0 | 3 | 0 | 1 | 2 | 1 | 0 | 7 |
| Total | 30 | 232 | 298 | 146 | 138 | 105 | 47 | 4 | 1000 |

*Table 2*  Complications in 1 000 consecutive abortions 1964–1968

| Complication | Number |
| --- | --- |
| Perforation of uterus (definite) | 3 |
| Perforation of uterus (suspected) | 1 |
| Pyrexia (antibiotics given) | 32 |
| Post-operative chest infection | 5 |
| Urinary-tract infection | 6 |
| Established intrauterine infection | 1 |
| Re-admitted with pelvic infection | 5 |
| Needing 2nd curettage within 48 hours | 16 |
| Re-admitted for prolonged, heavy bleeding | 4 |
| Needing 2nd injection of utus paste | 3 |
| Failure of utus paste followed by hysterotomy | 1 |
| Burst abdomen after hysterotomy | 1 |
| Persistent bleeding necessitating left oophorectomy during hysterotomy and sterilisation | 1 |
| Social or emotional problems | 2 |

the view of my family-practitioner colleagues who were well aware of the magnitude of the problem. Thus, my patients were a selected group being only those in whom complications or pain-intolerance had necessitated hospital admission; clearly there may have been local abortionists practising so successfully that I never had cause to suspect their existence. It must also be remembered that even of those patients who were admitted, there were undoubtedly many who claimed falsely that their abortion was spontaneous; it was only during the year 1965 that I made a really determined effort to discuss confidentially the problem with each one.

Of the 734 patients who admitted induced abortion to me, 381 were married and 353 single. Only a little over 10% said that they had induced the abortion upon themselves and I would guess that some women would falsely claim to have done so in order to protect a husband or lover. I do not think that women who had in fact aborted themselves would have any motive to claim that someone else had so acted. In my experience drugs taken to induce abortion were mainly ineffective. In many cases the woman had taken some form of medication days or even weeks before the abortion occurred, usually quinine tablets or ergot extracts and purgatives (Table 3). She often believed the drugs had worked, but in such cases I generally formed the opinion that in fact the abortion was really spontaneous and classified it as such. Those women who did succeed in procuring abortion by taking quinine always exhibited fairly severe symptoms of toxicity, in particular tinnitus and hearing loss. Possibly the series is unrepresentative in that women who did successsfully abort themselves medically may well have been less likely than others to develop complications needing hospital admission.

Table 3 shows that 21 women claimed to have aborted following vaginal douching alone. Most of these women had douched themselves — 'as hot as I could bear it' — and possibly many had inadvertently forced some fluid through the cervix. I did apply the same test as regards timing and onset of symptoms of abortion and was satisfied that in these 21 cases the douching was causal. Intrauterine injections using a rubberball syringe was common and at that time there was a vogue for using a strong solution of potassium permanganate crystals dissolved in water and usually boiled. One local abortionist had access to a supply of utus paste and was therefore using the same technique as we were in hospital, although she tended to use it for even very early abortions; I strongly suspect that we admitted only a very small proportion of her cases. Toothpaste sounds an unusual abortifacient but at that time there was a brand on the market with a particularly suitable end, easily

*Table 3* Kingston experience of techniques of illegal abortion

| | |
|---|---|
| Drugs alone | 17 |
| 9 Quinine Tablets with purgatives | |
| 3 Ergot extracts with purgatives | |
| 5 Purgatives alone or with alcohol | |
| Vaginal douching only | 21 |
| (All self-administered) | |
| Trans-cervical injections | 218 |
| 36 Soap solution | |
| 30 Potassium permanganate solution | |
| 24 Utus paste | |
| 18 Toothpaste | |
| 16 Hypertonic saline (Brine) | |
| 4 Whiskey | |
| 4 Boiled water | |
| 76 Solution or paste unknown to woman | |
| Intrauterine instrumentation | |
| A Sharp | 86 |
| 6 Deliberate rupture of membranes at 16 weeks or more | |
| 12 Crochet hooks | |
| 4 Uterine sounds | |
| 1 Thin lead pipe | |
| 2 Surgical artery clamps | |
| 21 Fine ovum forceps (cord cut) | |
| 40 Unknown to woman | |
| B Introduction of soft foreign bodies into uterus | 116 |
| 31 Male rubber catheter | |
| 20 Nylon cord | |
| 12 Plastic-covered curtain cord | |
| 10 Multiple I U C D s | |
| 38 Other soft tubing | |
| 5 Material unknown to woman | |
| Dilatation of cervix and curettage | 6 |
| 5 With general anaesthesia | |
| 1 Analgesics only | |
| Technique totally unknown to woman | 270 |
| Total | 734 |

pressed into the cervix. One ex-midwife used to perform abortions using a properly sterilised fine ovum forceps introduced through the cervix. She would find the umbilical cord, pull down a loop and cut it. Pain and bleeding were the reasons her patients were admitted, not infection. Nylon cord was pushed through the cervix by one abortionist who always left a long length of the cord accessible and would remove it as soon as contractions were established. Only once did I actually see this cord, when the young girl had panicked due to pain and came into hospital with it in place. Another local practitioner had hit upon the idea of inserting several, usually five or six, Lippes loops in early pregnancy. An ex-dentist who used to give a general anaesthetic and perform a D & C finally had an anaesthetic death when aborting a foreign girl in, I think, 1973; he served a term of imprisonment for this.

Unfortunately, because of an over-enthusiastic regard for the need to preserve the woman's anonymity I have no way of relating cases to complications, and indeed I have no proper records of the complications which did occur. There were no fatalities during the years surveyed, but there were a number of cases of septicaemia, and three women suffered acute renal failure, one requiring transfer to a hospital with facilities for dialysis. Incidentally, contrary to the experience of others, we never encountered a case of infection with *Clostridium welchii*.

It is exceedingly difficult to estimate the mortality of criminal abortion because, in general, neither the numerator nor the denominator is much more than an informed guess. The medical profession has tended to say that criminal abortion is exceedingly dangerous, and indeed this belief was responsible, in England at any rate, for the medical establishment doubting the high numbers of criminal abortions estimated by the police, demographers and others, simply on the grounds that there were not as many deaths as they would have expected. In fact when an individual doctor has studied the problem he has nearly always come to the conclusion that criminal abortion is far safer than generally believed, and Mohr [3] quotes the well-known East Coast gynaecologist, Dr Denham, who had taken just such an interest, saying in 1840 'in abortions, dreadful and alarming as they are, sometimes it is a great comfort to know that they are almost universally devoid of danger'.

In England and Wales, since 1952 every death of a pregnant woman, or of a woman who has recently been pregnant, is automatically reported by the Registrar of Deaths, and is made the subject of a confidential enquiry carried out by an appointed group of gynaecologists who collaborate with the local community physician, and who enquire of every doctor, midwife and, if appropriate, every nurse who had been in professional contact with the woman at the relevant time. An assessment is then made of what are termed avoidable factors, these being errors of judgment, either by the woman herself or by any of her medical or nursing attendants. The value of these reports is that every enquiry is totally protected and its findings cannot, under any circumstances, be used in any legal action, so that all may freely admit to errors they feel they have made, or challenge the wisdom of others in their management, without fear of damaging a colleague or of reprisal. The system works well and the reports are published every 3 years, as shown in Table 4 [7]. It is very likely that these reports are comprehensive and cover all cases where death has followed any form of abortion.

It will be seen at once that the deaths from criminal abortion have been falling fairly steadily ever since the reports were started in 1952, but that with the introduction of a liberal abortion law in 1968 the fall accelerated dramatically. Probably the initial fall was primarily due to the fact that antibiotics had become available, not only to the medical profession, but also to criminal abortionists who were certainly using them widely by 1965.

Since we now possess the numerator of our fraction I would like to try and estimate the mortality of criminal abortion in England and Wales over the years 1961–1966. To do this we shall have to exclude the years 1967, 1968 and 1969 because we do not know which of the deaths resulted from criminal abortions performed before or after the law had been made liberal.

One technique would be to accept the official Government estimate of 100 000 criminal abortions per year which was made in 1967 and assume that it may be applied to the preceding six years 1961–66, during which time we have seen there were 165 deaths. This would give a mortality of 27.5 deaths per 100 000 abortions.

The second method is more subtle but possibly even less accurate. It depends upon the fact that the sudden increase in the number of legal abortions performed had virtually no dramatic effect upon our birth rate, so we must assume that legal abortions performed upon resident women merely replaced abortions they would have previously obtained illegally. As a broad generalisation the increased number of legal abortions between the six years 1970–75 as compared with 1961–66 can be taken to be equivalent to the

*Table 4.* Deaths from Abortion in England and Wales, 1952–54 to 1973–75: abortion deaths in triennial reports on confidential enquiries into all maternal deaths (7).

| Type of abortion | 1952–1954 | 1955–1957 | 1958–1960 | 1961–1963 | 1964–1966 | 1967–*1969 | 1970–1972 | 1973–1975 |
|---|---|---|---|---|---|---|---|---|
| Illegal | 108 | 91 | 82 | 77 | 98 | 74 | 38 | 10 |
| Spontaneous | 43 | 50 | 52 | 57 | 25 | 25 | 6 | 5 |
| Legal | 2 | 0 | 1 | 5 | 10 | 18 | 37 | 14 |
| Totals | 153 | 141 | 135 | 139 | 133 | 117 | 81 | 29 |

* Liberal abortion legislation came into force on 27 April 1968.

number of criminal abortions avoided, and we can say that the fall in the number of deaths corresponds. It has been estimated that a total of 106 930 therapeutic abortions were performed in the years 1961–66 [8], whereas during the years 1970–75, 605 334 resident women had abortions. Correspondingly we have seen that the number of deaths from criminal abortion had fallen from 165 in the first six-year period to only 48 in the second. Thus we have an apparent saving of 117 lives by avoiding 498 434 criminal abortions. The calculated criminal abortion mortality is 23.5 per 100 000. This calculation is open to many criticisms. For example, it takes no account of improved contraceptive usage, and assumes that criminal abortion mortality remained constant. However, if we assume that these two estimates establish the right order of magnitude for criminal abortion, then we can see that liberal abortion legislation does save lives, quite apart from the squalid guilt and morbidity which is inseparable from illegal abortion.

With regard to therapeutic abortion, Tietze has repeatedly demonstrated beyond dispute that the more advanced the pregnancy the higher the risk. The recent British experience (Table 5) confirms that this still true. For the three years 1975–77 the mortality for abortion at less than 13 weeks menstrual age was 0.96 per 100 000, but 7.73 per 100 000 for second trimester abortion [9].

Partly because there is no cost borne by the patient, the British National Health Service has always performed a large number of sterilisations concomitantly with abortion, and we have also in the past had an excessive number of hysterotomies and hysterectomies performed as abortion procedures (Table 6). Our overall experience shows that when compared with vaginal terminations these two operations are over fifteen times as dangerous.

Apart from showing some illustrated figures from the British experience, I have not attempted to assess the mortality of therapeutic abortion, but having looked at the British figures, I found one glaring discrepancy which I would like to present, but totally without explanation.

As Table 7 shows, the mortality from abortion from 1968 to the end of 1977 in Britain was 7.6 per 100 000 in our total experience of 1 184 154 operations. The majority of these operations were in fact performed in the private sector, that is by doctors not working in the National Health Service (N.H.S.). This included two large charitable organisations set up to enable women to obtain abortions at a reduced rate if they were unable to obtain the operation under

*Table 5.* Abortion statistics for England and Wales, 1975–1977

| Maturity | No. of cases | Deaths* | Deaths per 100 000 |
|---|---|---|---|
| <13 weeks | 311 111 | 3 | 0.96 |
| >13 weeks | 77 623 | 6 | 7.73 |

* 3 deaths occurred but maturity not recorded

the N.H.S., or to afford normal private fees. Astonishingly, one finds that the mortality for this period within the Health Service was 15.84 per 100 000 abortions, whereas it was only 2.11 per 100 000 for private doctors. At first I thought that the possible explanation might be that the Health Service was dealing with seriously ill patients, but in fact virtually all the deaths which have occurred have been due to 'avoidable factors' such as anaesthetic complications, haemorrhage, sepsis and shock. It has also been suggested that women possibly obtain abortions more quickly in the private sector, and for some women this is undoubtedly true but, on the other hand the majority of women seeking abortion privately do so only after they have failed to obtain it under the N.H.S., so that quite possibly these two factors are cancelled out,

*Table 6.* Abortion statistics England and Wales 1969–1977: deaths from vaginal termination and from hysterotomy and/or hysterectomy (combined figures).

| Year | No. of vaginal terminations | Deaths | Rate per 100 000 | No. of hysterotomies and/or hysterectomies | Deaths | Rate per 100 000 |
|---|---|---|---|---|---|---|
| 1969 | 38 948 | 4 | 10.3 | 12 845 | 11 | 85.6 |
| 1970 | 68 703 | 7 | 10.2 | 14 159 | 6 | 42.4 |
| 1971 | 110 498 | 5 | 4.5 | 12 482 | 6 | 48.0 |
| 1972 | 132 819 | 8 | 6.0 | 9 203 | 6 | 65.2 |
| 1973 | 134 069 | 1 | 0.7 | 6 041 | 2 | 33.1 |
| 1974 | 150 004 | 5 | 3.3 | 4 098 | 1 | 24.4 |
| 1975 | 127 281 | 2 | 1.6 | 2 482 | 0 | – |
| 1976 | 117 761 | 1 | 0.8 | 1 940 | 0 | – |
| 1977 | 121 165 | 3 | 2.5 | 1 560 | 4 | 256.4 |
| Totals | 1 001 248 | 36 | 3.56 | 64 810 | 36 | 55.55 |

*Table 7.* Abortion mortality in England and Wales from 28 April 1968 to 31 December 1977.

| Year | National Health Service | | | Private Service | | | Total | | |
|---|---|---|---|---|---|---|---|---|---|
| | No. of abortions | Deaths | Rate per 100 000 abortions | No. of abortions | Deaths | Rate per 100 000 abortions | No. of abortions | Deaths | Rate per 100 000 abortions |
| 1968 (part) | 14 560 | 3 | 20.60 | 9 081 | – | – | 23 641 | 3 | 12.69 |
| 1969 | 33 728 | 15 | 44.47 | 21 091 | 2 | 9.48 | 54 819 | 17 | 31.01 |
| 1970 | 47 678 | 14 | 29.36 | 38 887 | – | – | 86 565 | 14 | 16.17 |
| 1971 | 53 706 | 10 | 18.62 | 73 071 | 4 | 5.47 | 126 777 | 14 | 11.04 |
| 1972 | 57 086 | 13 | 22.77 | 102 798 | 2 | 1.95 | 159 884 | 15 | 9.38 |
| 1973 | 55 637 | 4 | 7.19 | 111 512 | 2 | 1.79 | 167 149 | 6 | 3.59 |
| 1974 | 56 320 | 5 | 8.88 | 106 620 | 2 | 1.88 | 162 940 | 7 | 4.30 |
| 1975 | 51 147 | 2 | 3.91 | 88 555 | 1 | 1.13 | 139 702 | 3 | 2.15 |
| 1976 | 50 774 | 1 | 1.97 | 78 899 | – | – | 129 673 | 1 | 0.77 |
| 1977 | 52 732 | 8 | 15.17 | 80 272 | – | – | 133 004 | 8 | 6.01 |
| Total | 473 368 | 75 | 15.84 | 710 786 | 15 | 2.11 | 1 184 154 | 90 | 7.60 |

and it is unlikely that this would explain the significant difference that exists. An explanation should certainly be sought and, so far as I know, the figures have not been assessed publicly.

REFERENCES

1    Cole M 'Abortifacients' for sale *Abortion in Britain*, pp 43–45 Pitman Medical, London, 1966
2    Narkavonkit T  Massage abortion in Thailand  *People* (I P P F , London) 6 (3)  30, 1979
3    Mohr JC  *Abortion in America*  Oxford University Press, Oxford, 1978
4    Beric BM  quoted by Potts M  Legal abortion in Eastern Europe  *Eugenics Rev* 59  232, 1967
5    Rhodes P  *Abortion in Britain*, pp 25–34  Pitman Medical, London, 1966
6    Diggory PLC  Some experiences of therapeutic abortion  *Lancet* 1  873–875, 1969
7    *Report on Confidential Enquiries into Maternal Deaths in England and Wales, 1973–1975* Table 5 1  HMSO, London, 1979
8    Diggory PLC, Potts M and Peel J  Preliminary assessment of the 1967 Abortion Act in practice  *Lancet* 1  287–291, 1970
9    *Abortion Statistics for years 1961–66 and 1970–75*  Office of Population Censuses and Surveys  HMSO, London

## 5. THE TRIMESTER THRESHOLD FOR PREGNANCY TERMINATION: MYTH OR TRUTH?

WILLARD CATES, JR. and DAVID A. GRIMES

The orgins of many clinical practices are hard to trace. Clinical impressions, based on uncontrolled observations, make their way through the academic hierarchy of teaching rounds on hospital wards, to departmental conferences in hospital amphitheaters, to polished presentations at international post-graduate courses and to published chapters in widely-quoted texts. Finally, they become accepted as full-fledged clinical tenets. Along this path-way of increasing clinical acceptability, these judgements frequently go un-challenged — especially if rendered by individuals with sufficiently impressive reputations. Even worse, the tenets can subsequently develop a self-fulfilling prophecy of their own either by influencing directions of scientific research or by blurring interpretation of conflicting data. Thus, weak or unsound hy-potheses acquire a scientific respect that should be reserved for knowledge [1]. In short, they become accepted as truth when they should still be considered myth.

Pregnancy termination techniques have a rich and varied mythology. In many countries abortion is still illegal, so that data necessary to evaluate existing clinical tenets are limited. For example, before induced abortion was legal in the United States, clinical recommendations regarding pregnancy termination techniques came either from large numbers of complications after non legal abortions or from small series of 'therapeutic' legally induced abortions performed on high-risk patients in hospitals. This information often resulted in recommendations which subsequently proved to be in-accurate. To illustrate, as recently as the 1960s, a noted gynecology textbook advised hysterotomy for all abortions at 13 or more weeks gestation, bed rest for 4–7 days after abortion by curettage, and delay 'for as long as possible' before a second attempt to complete an incomplete abortion [2].

Fortunately, these myths have been made obsolete by comparative studies which have demonstrated safer alternative therapeutic approaches. Over the next 10 years, many of our current clinical tenets in abortion technology will probably become just as outdated.

The trimester threshold which limits pregnancy termination using instrum-ental uterine evacuation techniques to the first 12 weeks [3] appears to be another unsupported clinical myth. In this chapter we explore the historical foundation for the trimester myth, document the effect of the myth on

*M.J.N.C. Keirse et al. (eds.), Second Trimester Pregnancy Termination. All rights reserved.*
*Copyright © 1982 Martinus Nijhoff Publishers, The Hague/Boston/London.*

abortion practice, examine challenges to the myth based on clinical observations, and discuss the implications of abandoning this myth.

HISTORICAL FOUNDATION FOR THE MYTH

Obstetrical tradition customarily divides pregnancy into three equal parts, known as trimesters. The clinical basis for this separation is presumably empirical for certain important obstetric problems tend to cluster in each trimester interval [4]. For example, most spontaneous abortions occur within the first trimester of pregnancy, whereas most pregnancy-induced hypertension becomes clinically evident during the third trimester.

Landmarks in fetal development probably contributed very little to the trimester tradition. The skeletal system begins with the first sign of cartilage formation at approximately 5 weeks gestation [5]. This becomes progressively transformed into a bony matrix which subsequently calcifies. At about 8 weeks, the 'embryo' takes on human likeness: depending on the text, between 8 and 12 weeks, it evolves into a 'fetus.' Ossification of the skull begins in the fourth month, thus creating an embryologic point which hinders the evacuation of fetal tissue.

The occurrence of 'quickening' apparently has less association with a trimester than a semester approach. The first perception of fetal movement by the pregnant woman usually occurs near the midpoint of gestation, somewhere between 16 and 20 weeks of pregnancy [4]. Early common law in England and America did not formally recognize the existence of a fetus until it had quickened [6]. Thus this concept probably did not contribute to the formation of the trimester threshold.

Restrictive abortion legislation itself may have enhanced the development of the trimester threshold. Any complications occurring after illegal abortions exposed the participants to potential criminal litigation. Because uterine evacuation procedures become more dangerous as the length of pregnancy increases, practitioners protected themselves by setting a gestational age limit above which they would not perform the more hazardous procedures. Following obstetric tradition, a convenient point for this threshold was the end of the first trimester.

As induced abortion became legalized, the clinical tenet which had originated in obstetric empiricism and been adopted into illegal abortion practices became promulgated by those performing legal abortion. Initial research into the techniques and safety of legal abortion tended to reinforce, rather than challenge, the trimester myth. For example, the landmark report in the United States on suction curettage emphasized that vacuum aspiration alone was not adequate to evacuate the uterus after 12 weeks gestation [7]. However, the authors confined the internal diameter of the early suction cannulas to 12 mm, and they did not consider the supplemental use of ovum forceps or sharp curettage. Later reports by Stubblefield and his associates [8] have demonstrated the efficacy of larger-bore suction cannulas for evacuating uterine contents in pregnancies through 16 weeks gestation. Perhaps premature acceptance of the trimester concept limited technological development of suction cannulas only up to sizes of 12 mm, thus creating a self-fulfilling prophecy for the trimester myth.

Early observational studies of legal abortion morbidity also contributed to the trimester myth [9–11]. Although some of these investigations contained data which showed that instrumental uterine evacuation procedures after 12 weeks could be performed more safely than instillation procedures, they focused largely on the safety of suction curettage procedures performed *before* 12 weeks, and emphasized the advancing risks as gestational age increased primarily within the first trimester. By aggregating abortion methods into those performed before 12 weeks and those after, a false impression was created that all procedures performed in the later interval were quantum-levels more dangerous than those in the early interval.

Likewise, the trimester myth also influenced inferences based on analysis of specific abortion complications. For example, Conger and associates observed a marked increase in the rate of perforation at gestational ages beyond 12 weeks [12]. However, the numbers used to calculate these rates were small, and the denominators were estimates. Subsequent findings have indicated that underestimation of the actual length of pregnancy appears to be a more important factor in causing perforations than the gestational age [13]. Again, the myth of a trimester threshold affected the conclusions which were initially drawn.

Finally, in the United States the trimester threshold myth was incorporated into law. Faced with the large body of scientific data which artificially dichotomized abortions into first and second trimester procedures, in 1973 the Supreme Court ruled that states could regulate abortion services during the second trimester 'in the interest of the woman's health' [14]. This decision led many states to require that all second trimester abortion procedures be performed in hospitals.

To summarize, the historical foundation for the trimester myth appears rooted in subjective impressions which then became reinforced by objective measures limited in their conceptual approach. Analyzed differently, these data could have challenged the trimester myth. Obstetric traditions dividing pregnancy into trimesters became a convenient dividing line for illegal abortionists fearing criminal prosecution. This heritage was adopted during the early years of legally induced abortion, and the myth became supported by combinations of technical developments, analytic approaches, and judicial decisions.

44

Clinical practice based on the trimester threshold myth theoretically limited instrumental uterine evacuation procedures to gestations of 12 weeks or earlier. Thus, women requesting induced abortion at 13 weeks were forced to wait about 1 month to allow for transabdominal intra-amniotic instillation procedures. Consequently, in the United States far fewer abortions than expected were performed between 13 and 16 weeks — the so-called 'grey zone" of abortion practice — and many more than expected were performed after the 17th week (Fig. 1).

This skewed distribution was not indicative of the gestational age at which women initially request their abortions, but rather was an artefact of clinical practice based on the trimester myth. The distribution of abortions at earlier gestational ages fits an exponential curve. Extrapolating this curve beyond 12 weeks gestation forms a projected distribution showing abortions that would be performed if there were no 'grey zone' (Fig. 1). Most of the abortions performed at 17 weeks or later (shaded area on the right) would have been

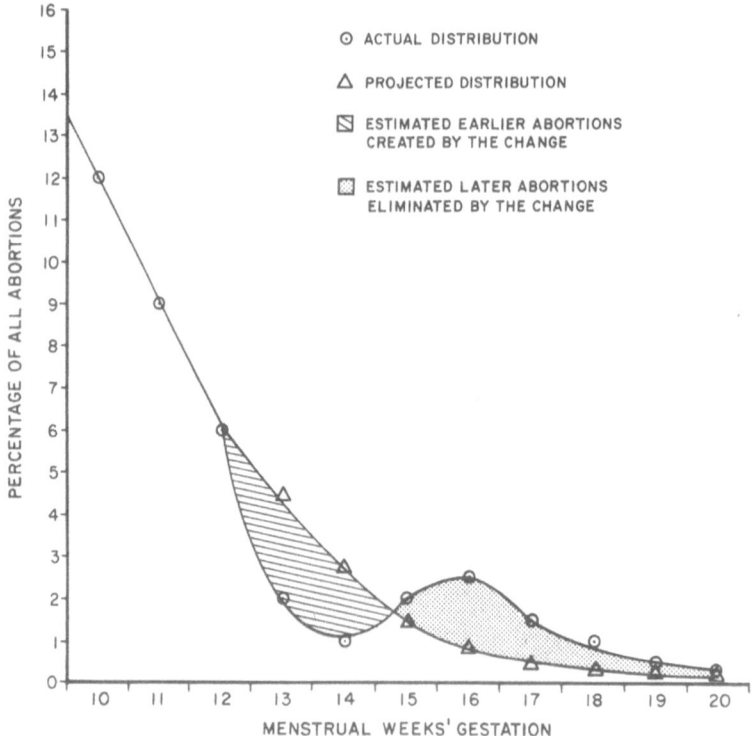

*Fig 1* Actual distribution of abortions and projected distribution without any delay in the 13 to 16-week interval, by gestational age (U S , 1975)

performed at 13 to 16 weeks (shaded area on the left) if no delay had been required. If abortions were performed when requested, about 80% of those performed at 17 weeks or later would be done earlier.

The 'grey zone' produced by the trimester threshold myth increased the mortality, morbidity, psychologic sequelae, and costs of abortion procedures performed at 13 weeks gestation or later. Regarding mortality, adherence to the 12-week threshold increases the risk of death for women requesting abortions at later gestations. For example, instillation of hypertonic saline has a death-to-case rate of 15.5 per 100 000 procedures, compared to that of dilatation and evacuation (D&E) after 12 weeks of 8.3 per 100 000 procedures [15]. Because the risk of death is directly related to gestational age, the death-to-case rate for D&E is lower (6.7 per 100 000) at 13–15 weeks gestation than at 16 weeks gestation or later (13,4 per 100 000). Thus, delays imposed by the 'grey zone' more than double the risks of death from abortion.

The psychological effect of the trimester threshold myth is also substantial. Waiting through the 'grey zone' prolongs the emotional turmoil that frequently surrounds unwanted pregnancies. Furthermore, selection of an instillation technique commits the woman to the psychologic trauma of long and uncomfortable labor [16]. Instillation procedures also involve the added emotional stress of her viewing the fetus at the time of expulsion; this experience has been reported to precipitate severe psychiatric reactions [17].

In addition to its medical risks, the trimester threshold is also expensive. If the 'grey zone' concept is followed, instillation procedures performed in hospital settings are three times more costly than suction curettage in clinics [18]. However, even most facilities performing D&E procedures after 12 weeks use the trimester threshold myth as a basis for setting fees; uterine evacuation procedures at 12 or more weeks cost one fee, whereas those at 13 or more weeks cost a larger fee, usually twice as much [19]. Thus although some abortion providers have abandoned the trimester threshold in their specific abortion *practices*, they have retained it in their *fee system*.

Finally, the trimester threshold myth focused abortion research on improving the *safety* of instillation abortion techniques, rather than questioning their need. Many of the initial investigations dealing with analogues of prostaglandins were directed toward second trimester instillation abortions, rather than examining their possible uses earlier in gestation. Likewise, research on the safety of saline instillation focused on such topics as the use of concurrent oxytocin and laminaria, the interval between fetal expulsion and placental removal, and the mechanism of its association with disseminated intravascular coagulation. While reducing complications associated with instillation procedures is important, many *more* complications could have been prevented simply by abandoning the trimester myth.

CHALLENGES TO THE MYTH

Gradually an increasing body of clinical experience and scientific observations created a reality which undermined the trimester threshold myth. The definition of what constituted a 'trimester' was never adequately addressed either in medical texts or judicial decisions. Moreover, the measures of gestational age are not consistent among available reports of abortion procedures. For example, length of gestation can be measured either from the onset of the last menstrual period (i.e. 'menstrual weeks') or from the estimated date of conception (i.e. 'ovulatory weeks', which is approximately 2 weeks less than menstrual weeks. Moreover, whether the dates are calculated in either ordinal or cardinal terms also affects reproductive age by one week. For example, the 13th menstrual week of pregnancy (i.e. ordinal) is 12 weeks after the last menstrual period (i.e. cardinal).

These difficulties in defining length of pregnancy have practical clinical applications (Table 1). For example, if a clinician refers a patient for an abortion who is '12 weeks pregnant', depending on whether her or his frame of reference was menstrual or ovulatory weeks, and ordinal or cardinal terms, the actual length of pregnancy could be anywhere from 77 days (i.e. first day of the 12th menstrual week) to 104 days (i.e. the last day of having completed 12 ovulatory weeks) amenorrhea. To complicate matters, if the clinician's estimate includes a range of weeks, such as '11–12 weeks pregnant', the interval of days amenorrhea would even be wider (i.e. 70–104 days).

Thus, the term 'trimester' lacked adequate definition for the practicing clinicians [3]. If the first trimester was interpreted to mean the first third of an anticipated 40 week pregnancy, then the first trimester extended $13\frac{1}{3}$ weeks from the last menstrual period. Alternatively, if the first trimester was interpreted to mean the first third of an expected 38 week pregnancy from the presumed date of conception, then the first trimester extends approximately $12\frac{2}{3}$ weeks from the presumed date of fertilization, or $14\frac{2}{3}$ weeks from the last menstrual period.

Besides the complexities of *defining* the trimester, the methods of *estimating* gestational age are at best an imperfect art. Menstrual dates are rarely recorded in a systematic fashion by many women, and thus memory failures are possible. Light vaginal bleeding early in pregnancy may be interpreted by some as a scanty menstrual period. Also, some women deliberately misreport their last menstrual period in an attempt to shorten the estimated length of pregnancy and thus qualify for the gestational age limitations of the particular abortion facility.

Physicians' estimates of gestational age from pelvic examinations are also subject to imprecision. Factors of obesity, tension in the abdominal wall, uterine sacculations, oligo- or polyhydramnios, multiple gestations and uter-

*Table 1.* Comparison of different dates and types of measurements on perceived length of gestation.

| Date and Type of Measurement | Perceived Length of Gestation | | | | | | | | | | | | | | | | | | |
|---|---|---|---|---|---|---|---|---|---|---|---|---|---|---|---|---|---|---|---|
| Ovulatory Ordinal Weeks | | | 1st | 2nd | 3rd | 4th | 5th | 6th | 7th | 8th | 9th | 10th | 11th | 12th | 13th | 14th | 15th | 16th | |
| Ovulatory Cardinal Weeks | | | | 1 | 2 | 3 | 4 | 5 | 6 | 7 | 8 | 9 | 10 | 11 | 12 | 13 | 14 | 15 | 16 |
| Menstrual Ordinal Weeks | | 1st | 2nd | 3rd | 4th | 5th | 6th | 7th | 8th | 9th | 10th | 11th | 12th | 13th | 14th | 15th | 16th | 17th | 18th |
| Menstrual Cardinal Weeks | | | 1 | 2 | 3 | 4 | 5 | 6 | 7 | 8 | 9 | 10 | 11 | 12 | 13 | 14 | 15 | 16 | 17 | 18 |
| Ordinal days Amenorrhea | 1st | 8th | 15th | 22nd | 29th | 36th | 43rd | 50th | 57th | 64th | 71st | 78th | 85th | 92nd | 99th | 106th | 115th | 120th | 127th |
| Cardinal days Amenorrhea | 0 | 7 | 14 | 21 | 28 | 35 | 42 | 49 | 56 | 63 | 70 | 77 | 84 | 91 | 98 | 105 | 112 | 119 | 126 |
| JPSA/CDC Intervals (menstrual cardinal weeks) | | | | | ≤8 (0–62d) | | | | | | 9 10 (63–76d) | | 11 12 (77–90d) | | 13 14 (91–104d) | | 15 16 (105–118d) | | 16 (119d or more) |

ine myomas limit accurate estimation. Moreover, the standard landmarks of uterine size taught in medical school, frequently based on 'citrus fruits', have their own inherent variability. One experienced clinician, examining women documented post-operatively to be more than 12 and less than 15 weeks pregnant, estimated pre-operatively that 24% were under 12 weeks while 12% were over 15 weeks [13].

Clinical experience with the latter situation, namely underestimation of length of gestation, led some clinicians to question the trimester threshold myth. When they attempted to terminate a pregnancy of 13 or more weeks, operators found that although later evacuations had more complications than earlier procedures, they appeared not only more practical but also safer than the later instillation procedures [13, 20]. Unfortunately, fear of peer criticism and of possible criminal prosecution in states where abortions after 12 weeks had to be performed in hospitals made these clinicians reluctant to openly challenge the trimester myth.

Thus, even while the scientific literature was espousing the trimester threshold myth, actual practice was evolving in a different direction. While some authorities [21] claimed that D&E was 'not widely used in the United States', the available data showed just the opposite. As early as 1974, D&E accounted for 65% of all abortions performed at 13 to 15 weeks and 11% of those performed thereafter. Therefore, even before the publication of data documenting the safety of D&E, many clinicians were using it to terminate pregnancies after the first trimester.

In addition, interpretations of abortion morbidity began viewing gestational age as a continuum, rather than artificially stratified into trimesters. After 8 weeks gestation, the risk of major complications appears to rise in a linear fashion, approximately 15–30% for each week of delay; there is no exponential increase which occurs after 12 weeks. A 2-week delay at 8 weeks gestation increased the relative risk of major complications at an even faster rate than a 2-week delay at 12 weeks gestation [22]. Thus, irrespective of the trimester threshold myth, *any delay* after 6 weeks increases morbidity. As indicated earlier, mortality trends support the same conclusion.

Since 1976, the literature has reflected what apparently had been the actual clinical practice. A growing number of case series reports and comparative studies have invalidated the trimester threshold myth. The most comprehensive of these studies was the Joint Program for the Study of Abortion, conducted under the auspices of the Center for Disease Control (JPSA/CDC). JPSA/CDC found that D&E procedures could be performed more safely than instillation of abortifacients [23]. Other recent studies have supported the JPSA/CDC findings. The complication rates have varied from study to study, because of the differences in technique as well as differences in data ascertainment and classification. Despite these variations, the case series reports indicate that D&E *can* be performed safely by experienced operators. The comparative studies indicate that D&E is even more safe than instillation of abortifacients. Thus, accumulating scientific evidence over the past 5 years has replaced the trimester threshold myth with the 'truth' of gestational age as a continuum.

PREGNANCY TERMINATION PRACTICES BASED ON TRUTH

Over the past 3 years in the United States, physicians apparently have increasingly rejected the trimester threshold. From 1974 to 1977, the overall proportion of pregnancies terminated in the 13–15 week interval increased from 37 to 44%, largely because of the increased number of D&E procedures. During these 4 years, the number of D&Es performed at 13–15 weeks more than doubled, and the percentage increased from 65 to 81%. Even after 16 weeks, the use of D&E procedures increased, from 12% in 1974 to 20% in 1977 [24].

The abandonment of the trimester threshold has also lowered the costs of the abortion procedure. Extrapolating from morbidity rates, abortion fees, and estimated treatment cost [25], we have projected that if instrumental evacuation abortions had been performed routinely in the 'grey zone' during 1975, the savings in overall abortion costs including both method and morbidity costs, would have been approximately $20 000 000 in the United States alone. This saving amounts to nearly two-thirds of the total estimated cost of *all* morbidity associated with legal abortions during 1975. It is reasonable to presume that the savings would be even greater in 1978.

Likewise, use of D&E procedures reduces the amount of hospital time required for later abortion procedures. Most D&E procedures are performed in a matter of minutes, rather than the hours required for instillation. Overnight hospitalization is usually unnecessary. In JPSA/CDC [23], women undergoing D&E procedures spent less time in the hospital (mean: 0.2 days) than women undergoing saline instillation (mean: 2.1 days). Efficient use of valuable bed space and staff time is becoming more important to both health agencies and consumer groups.

Using D&E procedures to terminate pregnancies later than 12 weeks also spares the woman much of the psychological trauma of instillation procedures. When interviewed 3 weeks after D&E experiences, women reported experiencing less pain and fewer negative emotional symptoms than did women who had undergone instillation [16]. Although D&E often involves greater emotional strain on the clinician and staff, use of the larger-bore cannula before 16 weeks [8] to evacuate products of conception would reduce for clinicians the emotional trauma of performing a procedure that is distasteful to them.

The abandonment of the trimester threshold has also saved women's lives. Since 1972, the overall death-to-case rates for legally induced abortion have been steadily declining in the United States, from 4.1 per 100 000 procedures in 1972–1973 to 1.3 in 1976–1977 [26]. We estimate that nearly 40% of this decline has been due to the abandonment of the trimester threshold. Since D&E procedures performed at 13–16 weeks gestation have markedly lower death-to-case rates *any* of the procedures performed thereafter, the switch to D&Es has contributed to the reduction in the overall death-to-case rate.

SUMMARY

The trimester threshold for pregnancy termination appears to have evolved from an accepted clinical tenet into the realm of outdated clinical myth. Over the next 10 years, many of our current clinical tenets in abortion technology willl probably become just as outdated. As scientists, we must keep an open mind regarding the need to continually evaluate the preferred approaches of providing medical care. We have made dramatic improvements, and many more will occur.

REFERENCES

1  Dykes MHM  Uncritical thinking in medicine  The confusion between hypothesis and knowledge  *JAMA* 227  1275–1277, 1974
2  TeLinde RW  *Operative Gynecology*, 3rd ed  pp  567–599, J B Lippincott, Philadelphia, 1962
3  Grimes DA and Cates W Jr  Gestational age limit of 12 weeks for abortion by curettage  *Am J Obstet Gynecol* 132  207–211, 1978
4  Pritchard JA and MacDonald PC  *Williams Obstetrics*, 15th ed  pp 246–247  Appleton-Century-Crofts, New York, 1976
5  Langman J  *Medical embryology*, pp  137–145  Williams & Wilkins, Baltimore, MD, 1975
6  Mohr JC  *Abortion in America  the Origins and Evolution of National Policy*, pp  3–5  Oxford University Press, New York, 1978
7  Kerslake D and Casey D  Abortion induced by means of the uterine aspirator  *Obstet Gynecol* 30  35–45, 1967
8  Stubblefield PG, Albrecht BH, Koos B, et al  A randomized study of 12-mm and 15 9-mm cannulas in midtrimester abortion by laminaria and vacuum curettage  *Fertil Steril* 29  512–517, 1978
9  Tietze C and Lewit S  Joint Program for the Study of Abortion (JPSA)  early medical complications of legal abortion  *Stud Fam Plann* 3(6)  97–124, 1972
10  Stewart GK and Goldstein P  Medical and surgical complications of therapeutic abortions  *Obstet Gynecol* 40  539–542, 1972
11  Nathanson BN  Ambulatory abortion  experience with 26 000 cases (July 1, 1970 to August 1, 1971)  *N Engl J Med* 286  403–407, 1972
12  Conger SB, Tyler CW Jr and Parker J  A cluster of uterine perforations related to suction curettage  *Obstet Gynecol* 40  551–555, 1972

13  Burnhill MS and Armstead JW  Reducing the morbidity of vacuum aspiration abortion  *Int J Gynaecol Obstet* 16  204–209, 1978

14  Doe vs Bolton, 410 US 179, 1973

15  Cates W Jr, Grimes DA and Tyler CW Jr  Safety of legal abortion  *Lancet* 1  198–199, 1980

16  Kaltreider NB, Goldsmith S and Margolis AJ  The impact of midtrimester abortion techniques on patients and staff  *Am J Obstet Gynecol* 135  235–238, 1979

17  Lipper S and Feigenbaum WM  Obsessive-compulsive neurosis after viewing the fetus during therapeutic abortion  *Am J Psychother* 30  666–669, 1976

18  Lindheim BL  Services, policies and costs in US abortion facilities  *Fam Plann Perspect* 11  283–288, 1979

19  Cates W Jr  For a graduated scale of fees for legal abortions  *Fam Plann Perspect* 12 219–221, 1980

20  Koplik L  Early midtrimester abortion by curettage  Presented at 13th Annual Meeting, Association of Planned Parenthood Physicians, Los Angeles, CA, April 7, 1975

21  Wolf JA and Rubinstein LM  Safety of prostaglandin F2a in abortion  *Am J Obstet Gynecol* 129  928–929, 1977

22  Cates W Jr, Schulz KF, Grimes DA and Tyler CW Jr  The effect of delay and choice of method on the risk of abortion morbidity  *Fam Plann Perspect* 9  266–273, 1977

23  Grimes DA, Schulz KF, Cates W Jr and Tyler CW Jr  Midtrimester abortion by dilatation and evacuation  a safe and practical alternative  *N Engl J Med* 296  1141–1145, 1977

24  Tyler CW Jr, Cates W Jr, Schulz KF, et al  Second trimester abortion in the United States  *Second trimester abortion  Perspectives after a decade of experience* pp 13–26 Berger GS, Brenner WE and Keith L (eds) PSG Publishing, Littleton MA, 1980

25  Von Allmen SD, Cates W Jr, Schulz KF, et al  Costs of treating abortion-related complications  *Fam Plann Perspect* 9  273–276, 1977

26  Cates W Jr and Grimes DA  Morbidity and mortality from second trimester abortion  A decade's perspective  *Second trimester abortion  Perspectives after a decade of experience* pp 163–178 Berger GS, Brenner WE and Keith L (eds), PSG Publishing, Littleton, MA, 1981

## 6. ASPIROTOMY FOR OUTPATIENT TERMINATION OF PREGNANCY IN THE SECOND TRIMESTER

W. Beekhuizen, K.J. van Schie, D.A.F. van Lith, M. du Plessis, and M.J.N.C. Keirse

The early part of the second trimester of pregnancy is traditionally recognized as a difficult period for the termination of pregnancy. Elsewhere (Cates and Grimes, chapter 5) it has been described as the 'grey zone', which has been responsible for an increasing delay and its ensuing risks in the termination of pregnancy. Whereas the amniotic cavity is not sufficiently developed to facilitate the application of intra-amniotic instillation techniques, placental expansion and the larger foetal parts hamper evacuation of the uterus by simple vacuum aspiration. Hence, when uterine evacuation is deemed to be necessary at this period of gestation a classical dilatation and evacuation technique (D&E) is usually resorted to, unless prostaglandins or prostaglandin analogues are available. Not infrequently classical D&E techniques require forceful dilatation with its possible consequence of cervical incompetence and may lead to possibly serious surgical complications. Therefore, as with the use of prostaglandins, hospitalisation is generally considered to be necessary. Altogether, it has led some to totally avoid termination of pregnancy at this period of gestation (Cates and Grimes, chapter 5).

The technique of aspirotomy was developed in Leiden [1], especially for the purpose of being able to deal with this period of gestation. The term *aspirotomy* is a contraction of the words *aspir*ation and embry*otomy* of which it combines the salient features. Fundamental to the concept of aspirotomy is that complete emptying of the uterine cavity must be possible without excessive dilatation of the cervix. For this purpose some of the principles of both vacuum aspiration and dilatation and evacuation were combined, and appropriate technical tools were developed.

It is the purpose of this chapter to examine whether aspirotomy can be considered as a safe and convenient procedure for outpatient termination of pregnancy in the early part of the second trimester. Furthermore, attention will be paid to some details of the procedure and its application that are of importance to those who intend to practise this technique. We shall therefore examine each of the steps in this procedure while drawing attention to their possible implications and our results.

*M.J.N.C. Keirse et al. (eds.), Second Trimester Pregnancy Termination. All rights reserved.*
*Copyright © 1982 Martinus Nijhoff Publishers, The Hague/Boston/London.*

Before discussing the various aspects of aspirotomy, a brief outline of the overall procedure is given here. After the woman is placed in the lithotomy position, 0.15 mg ergometrin is injected intravenously to assist uterine contraction. After local disinfection, about 30 ml of a solution of lignocaine 1% and epinephrine (adrenaline) 1: 200 000 is injected in and around the cervix. The cervical canal is then dilated by inserting overlapping sizes of Hawkin-Ambler tapered lightweight uterine dilators. Gentle handling of these instruments gives minimal trauma, especially since 10 mm dilatation is usually sufficient. A flexible plastic suction canula (10 mm) is introduced and the amniotic liquor aspirated. Then the aspirotomy forceps is inserted in closed position into the uterine cavity up to the uterine fundus, withdrawn about 1 cm and opened widely, so that the uterine content will fall between the jaws. Gently the forceps is closed and by manoeuvring it, the operator makes sure that no part of the uterine wall is caught. The bigger foetal parts are crushed and evacuated, as well as the placental tissues. If the products of conception are not easily obtained, suction is reapplied to manoeuvre the parts beyond reach in front of the ostium where they can more easily be caught and removed. A gentle check curettage is then performed with an 8 or 10 mm Evans sharp curette to assure complete evacuation. The procedure is finalised by vacuum aspiration with a 6 mm cannula, following which the patient is walked to her bed, where she is observed for another 1–2 hours before discharge. All products of conception are examined to confirm completeness and all relevant details are recorded in the patient's data sheets.

*Anaesthesia*

For an outpatient procedure local rather than general anaesthesia is essential. However, since aspirotomy cannot be performed in as short a time as a simple vacuum aspiration, anaesthesia needs to be of slightly longer duration to compensate for an operation time of 10–30 minutes. Moreover the procedure requires several instrumental manipulations through the cervical canal. To ensure adequate anaesthesia we therefore complement the traditional paracervical block of vacuum aspiration with intracervical injection of the local anaesthetic (Fig. 1). No sedation is used.

In practice the procedure consists of the injection of 1 ml of the anaesthetic in the anterior part of the cervix to allow painless application of a cervical tenaculum, followed by 5 ml paracervically at 4 and at 8 o'clock, followed by deep injection with an ordinary intramuscular needle into the cervical tissue of another 20 ml divided over 4 spots at 2, 5, 7 and 10 hours respectively (Fig.

54

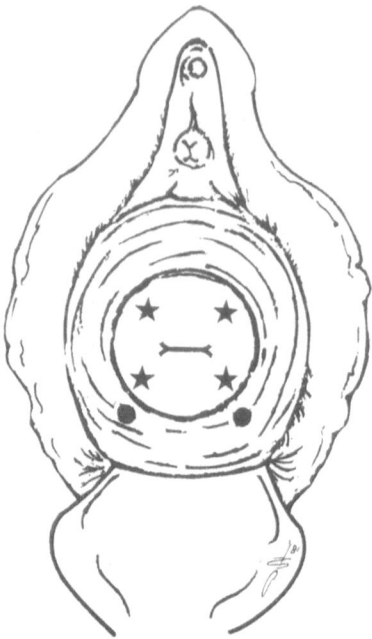

*Fig. 1*. Positions for the paracervical (black dots) and intracervical (asterisks) administration of the local anaesthetic.

1). These intracervical injections are rendered painless by the preceding paracervical anaesthesia.

The local anaesthetic used is a 1% solution of lidocaine (lignocaine, xylocaine) to which epinephrine (adrenaline; 1:200 000) is added [2]. Immediately after administration of the anaesthetic there is a general adrenaline effect (tachycardia, tremor, pallor) of which the woman should be warned in advance. This effect is maximal a few minutes after the injection and decreases rapidly thereafter. Dramatic changes in pulse rate or blood pressure have not been observed and in several thousands of cases we have experienced no serious ill effects of adrenaline at this low dosage. On the contrary, the addition of adrenaline is believed to have several advantages. Firstly, the maximal allowed dose of lidocaine increases with 150% to 500 mg, while the ensuing vasoconstriction ensures a longer local retention of the anaesthetic and a lower peak level in the circulation. Secondly, vasoconstriction of the branches of uterine arteries reduces uterine and placental blood flow. This effect, which can be observed during laparoscopy by acute pallor of the uterus provoked by the administration of the local anaesthetic, limits loss of blood during the procedure. Thirdly, the patient's circulation is supported by adrenaline to the extent that otherwise frequently occurring tendencies of bradycardia and collapse, due to the vagal stimulation provoked by the procedure, are not observed. Routine premedication with atropine is therefore not necessary. Occasionally however there may still be a vagal reaction at the end of the procedure, or shortly after its completion in which case intravenous atropine can still be administered.

*Dilatation*

In any vaginal procedure, the degree of cervical dilatation that is required is dependent on both the size of the products of conception that need to be delivered and the diameter of the instruments used to achieve that evacuation. For instance most ring forceps or ovum forceps used for the classical dilatation and evacuation procedures have a diameter of at least 13 mm and therefore require a cervical dilatation well in excess of 12 mm. In aspirotomy the degree of cervical dilatation can be greatly reduced by the combined evacuation procedure described below and by the use of aspirotomy forceps with various diameters. The cervix is therefore mechanically dilated only as far as required for the subsequent evacuation procedure or until increasing cervical resistance is felt, whichever occurs first. To feel the degree of cervical resistance adequately, it is essential to use tapered, lightweight dilators, such as the hollow stainless steel Hawkin-Ambler dilators, which are available in overlapping sizes (Fig. 2). In our experience these dilators are far superior to the classical Hegar dilators for this purpose.

Although most studies on D&E procedures do not state the degree of cervical dilatation that is needed, it can be appreciated from Table 1 that aspirotomy requires a lesser degree of cervical dilatation than most other evacuation procedures. Of 762 nulliparous women who underwent aspirotomy for termination of pregnancy in the second trimester in 1979, only 12.5% required a mechanical dilatation in excess of 10 mm. This implies that most procedures can be performed with the same degree of cervical dilatation which some consider to be appropriate [3, 4] or even necessary [5] for vacuum aspiration in the first trimester.

It is useful to realize that the cervix undergoes substantial changes during pregnancy. The cervix of the non-pregnant subject is firm and rigid; in-

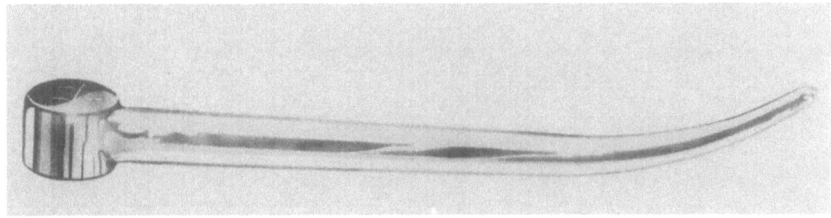

*Fig. 2* Hawkin-Ambler tapered cervical dilator (drawn by P Wiegman)

*Table 1* Cervical dilatation for the termination of pregnancy by aspirotomy at gestational ages of 14 weeks or more

| Reproductive history (all patients in 1979) | No of patients | No dilated > 10 mm | Percentage dilated ≤ 10 mm |
|---|---|---|---|
| Nulliparous and primigravid | 660 | 82 | 87 6 |
| Nulliparous but not primigravid | 102 | 13 | 87 2 |
| Parous | 467 | 97 | 79 2 |
| Total | 1229 | 192 | 84 3 |

strumental dilatation requires force and may result in injury. In pregnancy the cervix usually becomes increasingly soft and compliant. The altered physical condition of the cervix has been well described, mainly in relation to late pregnancy and the onset of labour [6], but the changes are not limited to that period of gestation. From early in pregnancy there is an increasing softening of the cervical tissue which is demonstrated by the fact that resistance to the intracervical administration of the local anaesthetic decreases with advancing gestational age. It is probably the increasing compliance of the cervix that is responsible for the gradual disappearance of the differences in cervical resistance and dilatation between nulliparae and multiparae with advancing gestational age (Fig. 3). At the lower gestational ages cervical resistance is far greater in nulliparous than in multiparous women. If due attention is given to these changes and differences in cervical resistance, they will have several implications for the degree of mechanical dilatation. In early terminations, dilatation will generally need to be less in nulliparous than in multiparous

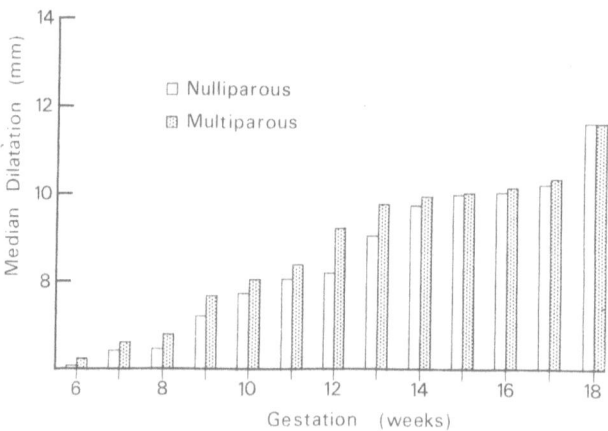

*Fig 3* Median cervical dilatation in relation to gestational age for all terminations of pregnancy by vacuum aspiration ( < 14 weeks) or aspirotomy ( ≥ 14 weeks, n = 1229) in 1979

women, a difference which is most marked in the period of 12–13 weeks before cervical compliance further increases (Fig. 3). Particularly in this period of gestation it appears to be necessary to avoid forcible dilatation and to use instruments with a small diameter. The increasing compliance with advancing gestation implies that a high cervical resistance in a rather large uterus should not be overcome at all costs. On the contrary, the high cervical resistance indicates that there may be other reasons (e.g. fibroids) for the uterine enlargement and that the pregnancy is probably less advanced and therefore not in need of that excessive dilatation.

*Evacuation*

At the very onset of the procedure 0.15 mg ergometrin maleate (ergonovine maleate, Ermetrine® or Ergotrate® is given intravenously to reduce loss of blood due to uterine atony. This drug is not the more potent methyl ergometrin (Methergin®).

The evacuation is started by the introduction of an 8 or 10 mm (dependent on cervical dilatation) plastic suction cannula that was specially designed with an extra opening at the top and that is longer than the usual vacuum aspiration cannulae (Fig. 4). The amniotic fluid is thus aspirated at a negative pressure of 685 mm Hg. The umbilical cord usually appears at this stage. Dependent on the degree of cervical dilatation an 8, 9 or 10 mm aspirotomy forcepts (Fig. 5) is then introduced into the dry and contracted uterine cavity. The forceps is advanced up to the uterine fundus, withdrawn about 1 cm, and opened widely to allow the uterine contents to fall between the jaws. The forceps (Fig. 5) is then introduced into the dry and contracted uterine cavity. ensured that no uterine wall is caught. Contrary to what is the usual practice in D&E procedures, the attempt is directed at delivering the placenta first, in order to prevent both uterine atony and excessive loss of blood. To appreciate

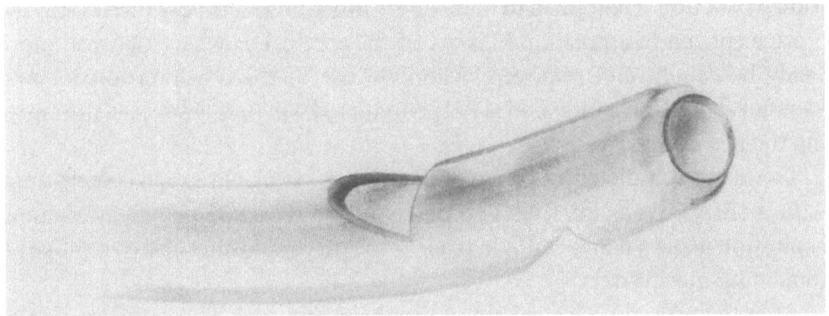

*Fig 4* Top end of the suction cannulae used for aspirotomy, the cannulae are slightly curved and have a length of 35 cm (drawn by P Wiegman)

58

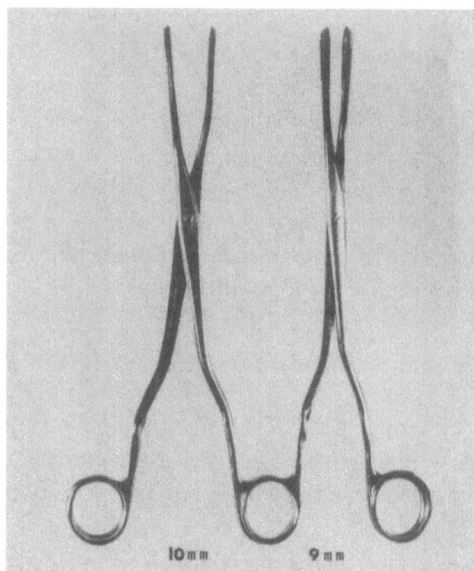

*Fig. 5.* Aspirotomy forceps.

the difference between placenta and myometrium it is essential to use the instrument loosely and not to handle it too firmly.

In general, an aspirotomy forceps of 8 mm will be adequate up to 15 weeks of gestation, whereas the 9 and 10 mm sizes are appropriate up to approximately 17 weeks. Occasionally it may be advantageous to use a smaller forceps especially to twist some of the larger parts around and to evacuate these in the axis of the cervical canal. Similarly, with adequate experience it is possible to grasp the edge of a rather large part and to make it follow the forceps through the cervical canal.

With gentle applications of the forceps even larger foetal parts as well as the placenta are crushed and evacuated. If no foetal parts are obtained by the forceps, suction is reapplied to manoeuvre those products beyond reach in the uterine cornua to a position in front of the cervical os where they can more easily be caught and removed. Alternate use of the crushing forceps and vacuum aspiration gently and slowly conducted will finally succeed in emptying the uterine cavity.

To ensure completeness of the evacuation, a check curettage is performed with a sharp Evans curette. The procedure is then completed by vacuum aspiration using a 6 mm cannula to clear the uterine cornua and to remove all remaining uterine debris.

After the procedure loss of blood should be minimal. The patient is able to walk back to her bed for a further period of observation of 1–2 hours before returning home.

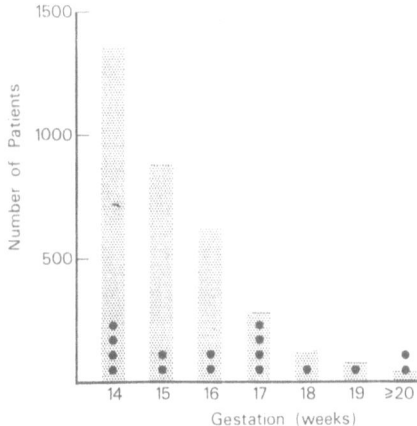

*Fig 6* The incidence of major complications (each dot represents one case) in relation to the gestational ages of 3370 women who underwent aspirotomy for termination of pregnancy in the years 1977–1979

COMPLICATIONS

*Immediate major complications*

In the years 1977–79 immediate major complications were encountered in 16 of the 3370 aspirotomies performed at gestational ages of 14 weeks or more. This incidence of 0.47% can be compared with the 0.6–0.7% major complication rate described by Tietze [7] for terminations at 13–16 weeks gestation in the USA during 1971–1975. However, when our complication rate is analysed in relation to gestational age (judged from the products of conception and expressed as the nearest week of amenorrhoea) it appears that there is a much lower incidence of complications at gestational ages of up to 16 weeks (0.28%; Fig. 6). Only one perforation occurred in 2854 aspirotomies at or below 16 weeks and all cases of haemorrhage (defined as a loss of blood of 500 ml or more) were due to delayed uterine contraction (Table 2). This is mainly due to an only partially removed placenta, which — even after administration of intravenous ergometrine — prevents timely contraction of the uterus and causes excessive venous loss of blood. Bleeding always stops after complete removal of the placenta and the subsequent administration of uterotonic drugs is therefore superfluous. Cervical injury from traction on the tenaculum was not considered to be a major complication, particularly since we use a Bierer toothed tenaculum.

At gestational ages of 17 weeks or more both the incidence (1.55 %; Fig. 6) and severity of complications increase markedly and their management often requires hospitalization (Table 2). In these cases haemorrhage was not always due to delayed contraction, but resulted also from uterine or cervical lacerations. From 17 weeks onwards the size and firmness of the foetal parts is such that the usual dilatation of 10 or 11 mm is often insufficient. Hence, mechanical dilatation to 13 mm or more and larger instruments are required with an apparent increase in the risk of complications and injury. This is a major reason for limiting outpatient management to pregnancies below 17 weeks gestation.

## Delayed major complications

Thus far information on the incidence of delayed complications is limited. In

*Table 2* Immediate major complications of 3370 aspirotomy procedures conducted in the years 1977 to 1979

| Weeks of gestation | No of cases | Type of complications* | Management of complications |
|---|---|---|---|
| Gestational age group of 14–16 weeks (n = 2854) | | | |
| 14 | 4 | haemorrhage | none |
| 15 | 1 | haemorrhage | none |
| 15 | 1 | cervical perforation | expectant, hospitalisation |
| 16 | 1 | haemorrhage | none |
| 16 | 1 | vasovagal collapse, convulsion | diazepam i v |
| Gestational age group of 17 weeks or more (n = 516) | | | |
| 17 | 1 | haemorrhage | none |
| 17 | 1 | uterine perforation | expectant, hospitalisation |
| 17 | 1 | uterine perforation | hospitalisation, laparoscopy, transfusion |
| 17 | 1 | cervical perforation, haemorrhage | hospitalisation, unilateral adnexectomy, transfusion |
| 18 | 1 | postabortum haemorrhage | expectant, hospitalisation |
| 19 | 1 | coagulopathy, haemorrhage, vasovagal collapse, convulsion | hospitalisation, transfusion |
| 20 | 1 | uterine perforation, intestinal laceration, haemorrhage | hospitalisation, uterine and intestinal repair, transfusion |
| 21 | 1 | haemorrhage | none |

* Haemorhage was defined as a loss of blood of 500 ml or more, unless specified otherwise or associated with perforation it was due to delayed contraction during the procedure

a consecutive series of 636 aspirotomy patients, who were instructed to return for a routine examination on the day after the operation, 525 women (82.5%) reported back for follow-up [1]. Postoperative pain (2.4%) and bleeding in excess of a normal menstrual period (2.1%) were the most common complaints. There was one case of excessive haemorrhage estimated at approximately 300 ml that required no treatment. One patient had a temperature rise above 38° C without signs of pelvic inflammatory diseases and was treated with antibiotics. None of the patients had felt a need to seek medical aid. Hence, it may be concluded that aspirotomy is suitable for outpatient termination of pregnancy below 17 weeks gestation.

There are no data as yet on complications that occur after a longer interval, i.e. complications occurring within one month after the procedure. Such a study is presently being conducted, but one should not underestimate the difficulties of assuring an adequate follow-up for this type of outpatient procedures and for patients who are predominantly of foreign nationality and from countries where these terminations are illegal. In other large studies [7] however, it has been demonstrated that the rates of delayed major complications, such as retained products of conception, infection, etc., differ little between patients with or without adequate follow-up.

*Late complications*

As discussed elsewhere (Berger and Keith, chapter 15), possible late complications include Rhesus sensitization and reproductive failure. Rhesus sensitization is entirely prevented by determining the blood type of all patients before aspirotomy and by the administration of anti-D gammaglobulin to all Rh negative women at the end of the procedure (Bennebroek Gravenhorst, chapter 16).

Reproductive failure after pregnancy termination is extensively discussed elsewhere (Rowland Hogue, chapter 19). On the one hand, this may consist of a failure to conceive that is most likely to relate to postabortal infection or to uterine or cervical trauma and/or its treatment. On the other hand, reproductive failure may consist of an adverse outcome, most notably spontaneous abortion or pre-term delivery in subsequent pregnancies. As discussed elsewhere (Rowland Hogue, chapter 19 = [8]), evidence on the realationship between induced abortion and the outcome of subsequent pregnancies is far from conclusive. Moreover, the mechanism by which induced abortions would affect gestational length in subsequent pregnancies is open to question, although cervical damage and subsequent cervical incompetence through forceful dilatation are currently the most favoured explanations.

Hulka et al. (9) found that increasing mechanical dilatation of the cervix results initially in an increase and then in a decrease of cervical resistance, which they attribute to a tearing of the internal os. In an admittedly small sample at early gestations, Johnstone et al. (4) found that cervices dilated to 10 mm or less showed virtually full recovery to normal size when measured at follow-up 6 weeks later, whereas cervices dilated beyond 12 mm frequently did not show full recovery. However, it is not clear to what extent these findings also relate to more advanced pregnancies in which there is increasing softening of the cervix; nor is it clear whether and to what extent such findings [4, 9] relate to the behaviour of the cervix in subsequent pregnancies.

Of potential interest with regard to aspirotomy in particular is the relationship between the degree and force of cervical dilatation and the subsequent risk of cervical incompetence and adverse outcome of pregnancy. If such a relationship could be duly substantiated, this might well imply that the attention to cervical resistance and limited mechanical dilatation gives aspirotomy a major lead over other procedures at similar gestational ages. At least in the Netherlands there are presently no indications that vacuum aspiration in the first trimester of pregnancy significantly affects gestational age in subsequent pregnancies (10). In as far as dilatations needed for aspirotomy are similar, this is likely also to apply to this procedure.

GENERAL CONSIDERATIONS

Before and during the procedure it is necessary to adequately inform the patient on each of the steps that are undertaken. She should be warned of the subjective symptoms that may be experienced. The effects associated with the administration of adrenaline have been mentioned above. Similarly, it should be pointed out that the procedure is usually followed by uterine cramps, which may in intensity exceed those of a menstruation but which hardly ever last for longer than 10–15 minutes.

Few procedures can be adequately performed without due attention to detail. Aspirotomy is certainly not an exception to this rule. Essential to the technique and particularly to maintaining a low complication rate are patience, gentle handling of all instruments and last but not least a certain degree of expertise. As with other procedures in the field of reproduction, e.g. laparoscopic sterilization, a rather easy and harmless intervention may quickly turn into an iatrogenic nightmare in the hands of hurried, careless and over-confident physicians. For this reason the operator should be seated and there should be no real time limit to the procedure. Like everyone else involved in the termination of pregnancy, the person performing aspirotomy may be exposed to emotional stress that can form a hindrance to careful and patient attention to detail. Rather than to ignore this factor, it is better to accommodate for it, for instance by limiting the number of sessions per week for each member of the medical and nursing staff. Another important consideration is to have a colleague at hand in order to ask for a second opinion on a rather unexpected uterine size or any other peculiarity instead of proceeding on good hope in these circumstances. This is of particular importance during the training process. Indeed, most complications arise at that time or when the trainee becomes too confident about the simplicity of the procedure. To avoid uterine perforation trainees should be well aware of the fact that a rather large uterus has a tendency to fall into retroversion during evacuation.

With the introduction of real-time ultrasound scanning it has become possible to further increase the safety of the procedure. Ultrasound is mainly used for measurement of the foetal biparietal diameter to ascertain a gestational age which is otherwise dubious. A foetal biparietal diameter of 42 mm is presently considered as the upper limit for outpatient termination of pregnancy by aspirotomy. Ultrasound scanning can also be an important aid during the training of operators, since they can then observe and check each of their actions on the real-time screen. The same principle can be applied when dealing with a uterine cavity with a rather unusual configuration. Ultrasound is also useful to check completeness of the uterine evacuation. Since there is no full bladder, it is then advisable to antevert the uterus with a suction cannula or aspirotomy forceps. Nevertheless, the best method to ensure completeness is a careful inspection of all products of conception. These can easily be identified when washed with and suspended in an ample volume of an aqueous solution.

As discussed elsewhere (Berger and Keith, chapter 15) adequate registration and record-keeping is essential for the constant evaluation of the technique and clinic performance and for maintaining a high quality of care.


CONCLUSIONS

In essence, aspirotomy carries the recognized advantages of first trimester terminations, i.e. a one-stage procedure, minimal cervical dilatation, local rather than general anaesthesia and outpatient instead of inpatient management, well into the second trimester of pregnancy. Nevertheless, there are limits to its application in that the risk of complications increases markedly with gestations in excess of 16 weeks or with foetal biparietal diameters in excess of 42 mm. If these limits are honoured, aspirotomy can be described as an inexpensive, exceptionally safe and convenient procedure for the termination of early midtrimester pregnancies.

64

REFERENCES

1 Van Lith DAF, Beekhuizen W and Van Schie KJ Complications of aspirotomy *Pregnancy Termination Procedures, Safety and New Developments*, Zatuchni GI, Sciarra JJ and Speidel JJ (eds), pp 193–205 Harper & Row, Hagerstown, 1979
2 Slome J Termination of pregnancy *Lancet* 2 881–882, 1972
3 Newton BW The art of abortion 1 Curettage of the pregnant uterus *Postgrad Med* 50 131–136, 1971
4 Johnstone FD, Beard RJ, Boyd IE and McCarthy TG Cervical diameter after suction termination of pregnancy *Br Med J* 1 68–69, 1976
5 Steptoe PC and Imran M Combined procedure of aspiration termination and laparoscopic sterilization *Br Med J* 3 751–752, 1969
6 Calder AA The management of the unripe cervix *Human Parturition New Concepts and Developments*, pp 201–217 Keirse MJNC, Anderson ABM and Bennebroek Gravenhorst J (eds) Leiden University Press, The Hague, 1979
7 Tietze, C *Induced Abortion 1979* p 82 The Population Council, New York, 1979
8 Keirse MJNC Epidemiology of pre-term labour *Human Parturition New Concepts and Developments*, Keirse MJNC, Anderson ABM and Bennebroek Gravenhorst J (eds), pp 219–234 Leiden University Press, The Hague, 1979
9 Hulka JF, Lefler HT Jr, Anglone A and Lachenbruch PA A new electronic force monitor to measure factors influencing cervical dilatation for vacuum curettage *Am J Obstet Gynecol* 120 166–173, 1974
10 Van der Slikke JW and Treffers PE Influence of induced abortion on gestational duration in subsequent pregnancies *Br Med J* 1 270–272, 1978

# 7. INSTRUMENTAL ABORTION IN THE SECOND TRIMESTER: AN OVERVIEW

DAVID A. GRIMES and WILLARD CATES, JR

Instrumental abortion in the second trimester of pregnancy encompasses a broad spectrum of technique, ranging from some of the oldest to some of the newest abortion methods. These instrumental methods can be divided into three broad categories; in decreasing order of safety, they are 1) dilatation and evacuation (D&E), 2) metreurynters and other traction devices, and 3) insertion of intrauterine foreign bodies. This chapter reviews the current status of transvaginal mechanically-induced abortion in the second trimester; pharmacologic methods, discussed in other chapters, and major operations are not considered.

## INCIDENCE

Although data are scarce, instrumental methods of second trimester abortion probably account for large numbers of abortions worldwide. In the developed world, D&E has emerged as an important technique. In Canada (1976), England and Wales (1975), and the United States (1976), D&E was the predominant method used for abortions at 13–16 weeks gestation (67%, 78%, and 69% of abortions, respectively). At ≥ 17 weeks gestation D&E was used for 8%, 39%, and 13% of abortions in these countries, respectively [1]. The large percentage of abortions at ≥ 17 weeks gestation in England and Wales performed by D&E probably reflects both longer experience with and greater acceptance of this method in these countries [2–6].

From the United Kingdom and Europe the D&E method spread to the United States, where it is currently one of the two most frequently used methods of second trimester abortion. In 1977 D&E accounted for 39% of the abortions performed at ≥ 13 weeks gestation, compared to instillation of hypertonic saline (38%) or prostaglandins (17%) [7]. The predominance of D&E as a means of second trimester abortion is striking in light of traditional tenets [8] of American obstetrics cautioning against its use.

In Japan about half of their relatively infrequent second trimester abortions are performed with metreurynters [1]. Little is known of the use of metreurynters elsewhere. Throughout the developing world and in countries where access to legal abortion is restricted, insertion of foreign bodies into the

66

uterus remains a common means of inducing abortion. An epidemiologic investigation of abortion complications in Bangladesh indicates that of women who sustained complications, over half underwent insertion of a foreign body as the primary abortion method [9].

DILATATION AND EVACUATION

D&E is a generic term for second trimester operations involving dilatation of the cervix followed by evacuation or extraction of the products of conception. Hence, it may be thought of as an extension of first trimester suction curettage. This section reviews the English language literature on D&E, first that published from outside the United States and then that from within.

## D&E experience in the United Kingdom and Europe

Bierer and Steiner [2] of London and Prague respectively, published one of the earliest reports on D&E in 1971. They used Hegar dilators and laminaria (with one to three packings for 24 hours) to dilate the cervix. Thereafter, they performed a podalic extraction or forceps extraction to empty the uterus. Among 390 patients from 12 to ≥ 20 weeks gestation, rates of hemorrhage, perforation, and antibiotic administration were 0.2, 0.2, and 0.8 per 100 abortions, respectively. Despite these low rates of morbidity, the method described may require several days for abortion, multiple exposures to general anesthesia, and cervical dilatation to large diameters (30–40 mm).

In 1972 Slome [3] of London reported his two-stage procedure used with 50 patients 16–20 weeks pregnant. Using paracervical block with local anesthetic plus vasoconstrictor, he mechanically dilated the cervix to 15–17 mm in diameter, drained the amniotic fluid through a needle, inserted laminaria, and administered an ergot derivative. After 24–30 hours, he evacuated the uterus with a crushing ovum forceps. No complications were reported.

Davis [4], also of London, described his technique of D&E in 1972. With the patient under general anesthesia, he ruptured the membranes, drained the amniotic fluid, then avulsed the umbilical cord. No laminaria were used. After 24 hours, he emptied the uterus with forceps. The only complication reported among 'more than 500 terminations' (gestational ages unspecified) was hypofibrinogenemia (approximately 1 case per 100 abortions). Although no cases of infection were observed, this method has the potential disadvantage of leaving nonviable tissue in the uterus for 24 hours in the presence of ruptured membranes.

In 1973 Finks [5] of London described a one-stage D&E procedure. He used an intracervical block with local anesthetic and vasoconstrictor followed by mechanical dilatation of 13–20 mm. General anesthesia was apparently provided as well. He then used crushing forceps to empty the uterus. Among 'over 2 000' abortions from 14 to 20 weeks gestation, there was one suspected injury to the uterus and one death due to a post-operative sickle cell crisis.

Slome [6], writing again in 1974, reported that by that time he had performed over 70 abortions by his method at 17-22 weeks; complications were not mentioned.

In 1974 Van den Bergh [10] of Heemstede, The Netherlands, described the experience of his clinic with the Finks technique [5] in more than 1500 women. Details about complications are limited.

In 1979 Van Lith and his associates [11] of Leiden published a report of their D&E technique, termed 'aspirotomy'. This name indicates that D&E represents a combination of vacuum aspiration and embryotomy techniques. Similar to the method of Finks [5], aspirotomy features a one-stage procedure, local anesthesia only, and dilatation to relatively small diameters ($\geq 13$ mm for a 19-week pregnancy). Among 636 patients at 14–19 weeks gestation, the rate of immediate operative complications and complaints was 1.7 per 100 abortions. At 24-hour follow-up examination, the rates for hemorrhage and fever were both 0.2 per 100 abortions.

*D&E experience in the United States*

In the United States a variety of D&E techniques [12–28] are practiced (Table 1). The upper gestational-age limit for performing D&E abortions is currently unresolved; it ranges from 16 to 24 menstrual weeks gestation in reports from individual institutions. The use of sonography to confirm gestational age is not uniform; instead, its use appears to be more selective. In the United States, second trimester D&E abortions are performed in hospitals as well as freestanding clinics, depending on local regulations, which vary from state to state. In both types of facilities, however, D&E abortions are usually done on an outpatient basis.

Most American physicians rely on laminaria to dilate the cervix (Table 1). The usual duration of laminaria placement is 12 to 24 hours, although DeLee [16] and Hern and Oakes [21] customarily use sequential packings of laminaria in the manner of Bierer and Steiner [2]. Other physicians rely on mechanical dilatation of the cervix in a one-stage procedure.

Either local or general anesthesia is used for D&E abortions. Two types of local anesthesia are employed: paracervical block or intracervival block, as described by Finks [5] and Van den Bergh [10]. Local anesthetics given for intracervical anesthesia include chloroprocaine with epinephrine [12] and lidocaine with epinephrine [19].

Most operators use special ovum forceps, such as the Bierer, Sopher or Van

Table 1 Differences in technique of dilatation and evacuation among reported single institutions, United States

| Study | Latest gestation (wks) | Facility | Routine sonography | Dilatation method | Anesthesia | Equipment |
|---|---|---|---|---|---|---|
| Barr [12] | 21 | Hospital | No | Laminaria | Local | Sopher forceps |
| Berry and Peterson [13] | 19 | Hospital | For gestations ≥ 18 wks | Pratt | Local | Peterson forceps |
| Boyd [14] | 18 | Clinic | No | Pratt | Local | Special forceps |
| Burnhill [15] | 16 | Clinic | Yes | Laminaria | Local | Heavy forceps |
| DeLee [16] | 24 | Hospital | No | Repeat laminaria | General | Ring forceps |
| Glick and Sacks [17] | 24 | Hospital | No | Laminaria | General | Special forceps |
| Goodman [18] | 19 | Hospital | No | Laminaria | Either | Sponge forceps |
| Grimes et al [19] | 21 | Hospital | No | Laminaria | Local | Bierer forceps |
| Hanson [20] | 20 | Hospital | No | Laminaria | Local | Sponge forceps |
| Hern and Oakes [21] | 19 | Clinic | Yes | Repeat laminaria | Local | Bierer forceps |
| Hodari et al [22] | 20 | Hospital | No | Pratt | General | Ring forceps |
| Hubacker [23] | 24 | Hospital | No | Laminaria | Either | Large cannula / Sopher forceps |
| Kaltreider et al [24] | 20 | Hospital | No | Laminaria | General | Sopher forceps |
| Koplik [25] | 16 | Clinic | No | Laminaria | Local | Special forceps |
| Livingston [26] | 16 | Clinic | No | Hanks | General | Sponge forceps |
| Meadowbrook [27] | 20 | Clinic ≤ 18 wks | No | Laminaria | Local | Special forceps |
| Stubbefield et al [28] | 18 | Hospital | No | Laminaria | Either | Large cannula, Foerester forceps |

Lith forceps to remove the fetal tissues. Stubblefield and associates [28], however, in a randomized clinical trial found that a 15.9 mm diameter suction cannula adequately evacuated pregnancies to 16 menstrual weeks, thus obviating the need for crushing forceps. These authors commented that elimination of fetal dismemberment may make D&E more acceptable to physicians.

Administrations of oxytocic agents and antibiotics varies from institution to institution. Some physicians administer oxytocin during the operation to decrease bleeding and to provide a firmer uterine wall. Others, however, avoid oxytocics for fear of 'trapping' the fetal calvarium. Prophylactic tetracycline or doxycycline are sometimes given.

D&E appears to be the safest available method of second trimester abortion in the United States. As summarized in Table 2, many reports [12–13, 15–26, 28–35] have documented low morbidity rates for D&E, with major complication rates ranging from 0.4 to 1.7 per 100 abortions and total complications rates ranging from 2.8 to 10.2.

Studies comparing D&E and instillation techniques are more useful in evaluating the safety of D&E. We are aware of five prospective nonrandomized cohort studies (one single institution and four multicenter) and one randomized clinical trial that have compared D&E with instillation abortions. The conclusion of each study was similar: D&E seems safer than current abortifacients.

Kaltreider and associates [24] focused on the psychologic morbidity of D&E and instillation of prostaglandin $F_{2\alpha}$ ($PGF_{2\alpha}$) on patients and staff. They found that with D&E patients had less pain, guilt, depression, and anger than with $PGF_{2\alpha}$. On the other hand, they observed that with D&E much of the emotional burden of second trimester abortion was shifted from the patient to the physician.

The first large collaborative study of abortion complications in the United States, the Joint Program for the Study of Abortion sponsored by the Population Council [29, 30], found that the major complication rate for D&E at 13-14 weeks gestation (0.8 per 100 abortions) was less than for saline instillation at any gestational age (1.4–2.5). Similarly, the total complication rate for D&E at $\geq 15$ weeks gestation (7.9 per 100 abortions) was less than that for saline at any gestational age (21.0–29.5).

A multicenter study by the International Fertility Research Program [32] found that performing D&E abortions in the 13–15-week interval may be safer than delaying patients until 16 weeks or later for instillation of saline. The total complication rate for D&E at 13-15 weeks was 12.5 per 100 abortions, while that for saline instillation at 16-18 weeks was 10.6. The authors cautioned, however, that saline instillation appears to be associated with higher rates of serious complications, such as infections, pulmonary complications, and death.

Smith and his associates [35] in Hawaii reached the same conclusion as the investigators at the International Fertility Research Program [32]. They found that in the 13–16 week interval curettage methods had a total complication rate of 12.3–13.9 per 100 abortions, while saline instillation had a rate of 33.5. Thus, they concluded that D&E is the method of choice at 13–16 weeks gestation. Delays to ≥ 16 weeks gestation to allow amnioinfusion to be done are not medically justifiable.

The continuation of the Joint Program for the Study of Abortion, conducted by the Center for Disease Control [33], corroborated the earlier findings of The Population Council study [29, 30]. Comparing over 6000 D&E and 8000 saline instillation abortions at 13–20 weeks gestation, these investigators found D&E to be significantly safer. D&E had a major complication rate of 0.69 per 100 abortions, in contrast to 1.78 for saline instillation. Women who received saline also required treatments of complications significantly more often.

Because methodologic weaknesses in these studies might have accounted in part for the differences observed, investigators at the University of North Carolina [19] evaluated the safety and feasibility of D&E versus $PFG_{2\alpha}$ instillation in a randomized clinical trial. One hundred women thought to be 13-18 weeks pregnant were enrolled, and 50 were allocated randomly to each group. Subjects assigned to $PGF_{2\alpha}$ waited significantly longer to obtain an abortion, and significantly more of these women dropped out of the study. The total complication rates for D&E and $PGF_{2\alpha}$ were 6 and 34 per 100 abortions respectively, a significant difference. No major complications occured in the D&E group, in contrast to 3 in the $PGF_{2\alpha}$ group. All but two D&E subjects underwent abortion as outpatients, while all receiving $PGF_{2\alpha}$ were hospitalized one or more nights. Thus, the only randomized clinical trial to date confirms the findings of previous observational studies: D&E appears safer than instillation of abortifacients.

Mortality statistics from the United States support the greater relative safety of D&E compared to instillation abortions. From 1972 to 1977, D&E had an overall death-to-case rate of 8.3 per 100 000 abortions, compared with 14.1 for instillation of abortifacients [7]. Thus, the risk of death from a D&E abortion in the second trimester is higher than that from suction curettage in the first trimester (1.2 per 100 000 abortions) but lower than that from second trimester instillation techniques.

In summary, D&E appears safer, faster, less expensive, and more convenient than instillation abortions. No live births occur. On the other hand, D&E requires more technical facility and greater physician involvement in the abortion process. As with other methods, the potential long-term sequelae of D&E remain unknown. Existing data (Table 2), however, indicate that D&E is preferable to methods of abortion that rely on induction of labor.

*Table 2* Studies of dilatation and evacuation procedures, United States

| Study | Type study | Number of patients (weeks gestation) | Findings |
|---|---|---|---|
| Tietze and Lewit [29, 30] | Multicenter, prospective, cohort, non-randomized | N = 2734<br>2,317 (13–14)<br>417 (15+) | Complication rates increase with increasing gestational age Total complications for D&E less than saline at all gestations |
| Stewart and Goldstein [31] | Case series | N = 195<br>180 (13–14)<br>15 (15–16) | Complication rates increase with gestational age No comparison of D&E and saline complications |
| Brenner and Edelman (includes data from U S , England, India and Singapore) [32] | Multicenter, prospective, cohort, non-randomized | N = 338 (13–15) | Complication rates with sharp curettage through 15 weeks similar to saline at later gestations Suction curettage alone had higher complication rates than sharp curettage alone |
| Koplik [25] | Case series | N = 141<br>95 (13–14)<br>46 ( > 14) | No significant difference in complications by gestational age |
| DeLee [16] | Case series | N = 47<br>28 (14–16)<br>12 (17–19)<br>6 (20–22)<br>1 (23–24) | No major complications One minor complication of fever |
| Grimes et al [33] | Multicenter, prospective, cohort, non-randomized | N = 6213<br>5632 (13–16)<br>581 (17–20) | Major complications for D&E 60% lower than for saline instillation |

Table 2 (continued)

| Study | Type study | Number of patients (weeks gestation) | Findings |
|---|---|---|---|
| Hodari et al [22] | Case series | N = 2490<br>1144 (15)<br>1012 (16)<br>267 (17)<br>57 (18)<br>7 (19)<br>3 (20) | Major complication rate of 1 65/100 D&E procedures Total complication rate of 2 77/100 D&E procedures |
| Hern and Oakes [21] | Case series | N = 150<br>45 (13)<br>35 (14)<br>44 (15)<br>16 (16)<br>5 (17)<br>4 (18)<br>1 (19) | Mean blood loss 117 cm$^3$, mean operative time 10 minutes, one suspected uterine perforation, no major complications |
| Goldsmith et al [34] | Case series | N = 130<br>24 (14–15)<br>59 (16–17)<br>36 (18–19)<br>11 (20) | Complication rates with D&E similar to those found in JPSA/CDC Slightly higher rates for infection and retained tissue than JPSA/CDC |
| Goodman [18] | Case series | N = 50<br>17 (14–15)<br>22 (16–17)<br>11 (18–19) | No major complications One case of febrile morbidity |
| Livingston [26] | Case series | N = 6168<br>5896 (13–14)<br>272 (15–16) | Major complication rate of 0 58/ 100 D&E procedures Total complication rate of 7 4/100 D&E |

73

*Table 2* (continued)

| Study | Type study | Number of patients (weeks gestation) | Findings |
|---|---|---|---|
| Burnhill [15] | Case series | N = 568<br>207 (15)<br>348 (16)<br>6 (17)<br>6 (18)<br>1 (19) | Total complication rate of 10 2/100 D&E procedures Perforations 14 times more frequent with D&E after 14 menstrual weeks than before  Series based on underestimated gestations |
| Smith et al [35] | Multicenter, prospective, cohort, non-randomized | N = 721<br>696 (13–16)<br>25 (17–20) | Complication rates with D&E in 13–16 week range less than instillation procedures later |
| Stubblefield et al [28] | Case series | N = 73<br>21 (13)<br>20 (14)<br>20 (15–16)<br>12 (17–18) | No major complications  Larger cannula had greater blood loss at lower gestational ages, but faster and more complete uterine evacuation |
| Barr [12] | Case series | N = 900<br>48 3% (18–20) | Major complication rate 0 44/100 D&E procedures  Two uterine perforations |
| Glick and Sacks [17] | Case series | N = 1074<br>334 (≤ 15)<br>289 (16)<br>267 (17–18)<br>156 (19–20)<br>23 (21–22)<br>5 (23–24) | Major complication rate 0 55/100 D&E procedures  Five cases of DIC, one recognized perforation |
| Hanson [20] | Case series | N = 3123<br>819 (14)<br>673 (15)<br>465 (16)<br>281 (17) | Major complication rate of 0 2% |

*Table 2* (continued)

| Study | Type study | Number of patients (weeks gestation) | Findings |
|---|---|---|---|
| Berry and Peterson [13] | Case series | 332 (18)<br>246 (19)<br>200 (20)<br>21 (21)<br><br>N = > 5000 | Rate of uterine perforation <0 4/100, transfusion <0 1/100, infection 0 3/100 |
| Kaltreider et al [24] | Cohort, Non-randomized | N = 250<br>52 (14–15)<br>106 (16–17)<br>72 (18–19)<br>20 (≥ 20) | D&E was associated with greater comfort and less guilt, anger and depression than $PGF_{2\alpha}$ |
| Grimes et al [19] | Randomized clinical trial | N = 94<br>8 (≤ 12)<br>16 (13–14)<br>34 (15–16)<br>27 (17–18)<br>6 (19–20)<br>3 (≥ 21) | Total complication rate 6/100 D&E procedures, 34/100 $PGF_{2\alpha}$ procedures Significantly better compliance with D&E regimen, shorter hospital stay, fewer gastrointestinal side effects |
| Hubacker [23] | Case series | N = 224<br>51 (16)<br>45 (17)<br>39 (18)<br>31 (19)<br>24 (20)<br>13 (21)<br>10 (22)<br>6 (23)<br>5 (24) | Major complication rate 1 8/100 procedures, minor complication rate 3 6/100 procedures |

The metreurynter is an inflatable rubber device designed to apply pressure against the lower uterine segment. Described by Champetier de Ribes in 1888 in Europe and adopted thereafter by Japanese physicians, the metreurynter resembles an eggplant-shaped Foley catheter with a 100–300 cm$^3$ capacity balloon [36]. Indeed, a Foley catheter with a 75 cm$^3$ balloon has been used as a substitute for a metreurynter [37]. The device is sterilized, then inserted through a partially dilated cervix into the extraovular space. The distal end of the metreurynter is attached by a cord to an orthopedic traction device of 300 to 800 g at the foot of the patient's bed. Oxytocic drugs and antibiotics are routinely administered thereafter [36–40].

Dilatation of the cervix and insertion of the metreurynter can involve one or more steps. In the one stage procedure the operator mechanically dilates the cervix to a large diameter (12 to 16 Hegar) then inserts the metreurynter [36]. Alternatively, one may insert two or three laminaria for a period of 24 hours, remove the laminaria, then insert the metreurynter. As another option, the physician may use two serial 24-hour placements of laminaria followed by insertion of the metreurynter on the third day. Use of laminaria shortens the time the metreurynter must remain in place. With 24-hour pre-treatment with laminaria, the duration of metreurynter application ranges from 15 to 40 hours, while with 48 hour pre-treatment, the duration ranges from 5 to 24 hours [37].

Metreurynters induce abortion primarily by a mechanical effect; placental dysfunction and fetal death do not routinely occur [38]. Japanese authors speculate that distension of the lower uterine segment by the metreurynter bag increases the intrinsic myogenic activity of the uterus [36, 39]. In addition, use of the metreurynter increases the sensitivity of the uterus to exogenous oxytocin [40]. With the laminaria-metreurynter method, uterine contractility resembles term labor rather than that produced by instillation of abortifacients. Manabe and associates [39] observed that contractions were usually < 50 mm Hg in intensity and occurred at a rate of 2–5 per 10 minutes; uterine activity was usually within 200 Montevideo units.

The efficacy of metreurynter-induced abortions appears less than that of available alternatives. Analysis of the 953 cases summarized by Manabe [36] reveals a rate of abortion of only 86% (time unspecified) despite the common use of oxytocin augmentation [41].

Complication rates are difficult to evaluate. Despite the use of prophylactic antibiotics (unspecified), Manabe and Nakajima [37] reported a rate of fever ≥ 38° C of 7% among 230 patients; they noted a rate of retained placenta of 8%. In a series of 469 such abortions, other investigators reported a rate of fever ≥ 38°C of 1% and not a single retained placenta [37]. Although Manabe

[39] acknowledges that 'prolonged treatment with the metreurynter increases the chance of infection', he boldly claims that the metreurynter has been used widely in Japan '...for some 20 years, and no serious side effects have ever been reported.'

Advantages of the metreurynter method include the lack of need for amniocentesis and the applicability of the technique at any time during the second or third trimester of pregnancy. Disadvantages include prolonged abortion times and hospitalization, relatively low abortion rates, relatively high rates of fever, prolonged immobilization of the patient in bed, the requirement of oxytocic agents and antibiotics, and a very high rate of liveborn fetuses. Although still practiced in Japan as a primary method of abortion, the metreurynter should probably be used only as a secondary technique in unique circumstances. An example would be completion of a failed instillation abortion at a gestational age at which the physician would not feel comfortable using D&E and in a setting where newer prostaglandin abortifacients were not available.

INTRAUTERINE FOREIGN BODIES

Insertion of a foreign body into the uterus is one of the oldest and least desirable methods of abortion. This approach has traditionally played an important role in abortions initiated by women themselves or by other lay persons; even today the practice persists in the legal sphere in some locales [42]. This section reviews recent experience with catheters and bougies, balsa, and plastic coils.

A bougie is an elastic gum tube, 0.5–1.0 cm in diameter and 30–45 cm in length. After the tube has been sterilized, the operator inserts one or two bougies between the fetal membranes and uterine wall until the tips of the bougies lie at the fundus. He then cuts off the excess length of bougie and packs the vagina with disinfectant gauze to prevent expulsion. The ensuing labor generally expels the bougies. As with abortion by metreurynter, concurrent treatment with oxytocics and prophylactic antibiotics is common [36].

Mullick and associates [43] reported their experience with 50 patients who had one to three Mullick catheters inserted to induce abortion. Each patient received prophylactic antibotics during the abortion and for 4 days thereafter.

Other objects used to initiate abortion include pieces of balsa [43] and plastic coils [43, 44]. The 'super coil' is a plastic strip 35 cm long and 4.6 mm wide, which is wound into a coil approximately 3 cm in diameter. To insert the coil into the extraovular space, the operator draws the coil into an inserter (like an IUD inserter) then expels the device into the uterus through the cervix. The coil is supposed to resume its original configuration in the uterus then gradually unwind until its diameter is 5–10 cm. Several coils are inserted, then removed 12–24 hours later by means of strings attached to each. If the uterine contents have not been expelled by the time of removal of the coils, the operator evacuates the cavity with sponge forceps.

The effectiveness of foreign bodies in achieving abortion varies widely. Manabe's review [36] reports rates ranging from 71 to 100% with bougies in Japan. Mullick and associates [43] report a success rate of 70% with catheters, 82% with coils alone, and 81% with coils plus balsa.

Complication rates with foreign bodies are unacceptably high, although Manabe [36] asserts that rates of febrile morbidity are lower than with metreurynters. The report by Mullick and associates [43] included only complications requiring hospitalization, and hence lacks sufficient information to allow adequate comparison of complications. Nevertheless, two of 17 patients (12%) undergoing abortion by coils had serious complications: one with peritonitis despite prophylactic antibiotics and the other with hemorrhage requiring transfusion. Investigation of a cluster of morbidity related to use of coils in a city in the United States demonstrated a complication rate of 60% in 15 women, including one hysterectomy [44].

The risk of death associated with abortion by catheter placement is high. Three of 12 reported deaths from sepsis after legal abortion the United States from 1975 to 1977 followed placement of an intrauterine catheter [45]. Although the number of abortions performed by this method in the United States is unknown, we presume it is small.

The hazards of abortion by placement of intrauterine foreign bodies are probably greater in the developing world. The previously cited epidemiologic surveillance of abortion-related deaths in Bangladesh indicates that approximately 10 000 women die each year in that nation after such abortions, performed primarily by lay midwives [9].

The sole advantage of insertion of foreign bodies is that this method is probably simpler to initiate than alternative techniques. On the other hand, as with metreurynters, disadvantages are numerous including relatively low efficacy, a high percentage of patients requiring a second procedure, long abortion times (up to 15 days in one report [46]) and high complication rates, particularly with coils. Thus, inert foreign bodies are a relatively inefficient and hazardous means of abortion in the second trimester.

SUMMARY

Instrumental methods of abortion probably account for large numbers of second trimester pregnancy terminations worldwide. Available data indicate that D&E is preferable to abortion methods that induce labor  Metreurynters and other traction devices have relatively long abortion times and high rates of febrile morbidity  Hence, these techniques should be considered ancillary rather than primary abortion methods  Insertion of foreign bodies into the uterus is an inefficient and hazardous means of inducing abortion  Provision of safer methods of legal abortion to women throughout the world can minimize reliance on this archaic technique

## REFERENCES

1  Tietze C  *Induced Abortion  1979*  The Population Council, New York, 1979
2  Bierer I and Steiner V  Termination of pregnancy in the second trimester with the aid of laminaria tents  *Med Gynaecol Soc* 6  9–10, 1971
3  Slome J  Termination of pregnancy  *Lancet* 2  881–882, 1972
4  Davis G  Mid-trimester abortion  *Lancet* 2  1026, 1972
5  Finks AA  Mid-trimester abortion  *Lancet* 1  263–264, 1973
6  Slome J  Mid-trimester termination  *Br Med J* 3  631, 1974
7  Center for Disease Control  *Abortion Surveillance 1977*  Issued September, 1979
8  Grimes DA and Cates W Jr  Gestational age limit of 12 weeks for abortion by curettage  *Am J Obstet Gynecol* 132  207–210, 1978
9  Rosenberg M  Abortion mortality in Bangladesh  Presented at 29th Annual Epidemic Intelligence Service Conference, Center for Disease Control, Atlanta, GA, 1980
10  Van den Bergh AS  Abortion procured in the second trimester of pregnancy  *Medisch Contact* 29  1555–1560, 1974
11  Van Lith DAF, Beekhuizen W and van Schie KJ  Complications of aspirotomy (AT) a modified dilatation and curettage procedure for terminating early second trimester pregnancies  In  *Pregnancy Termination  Procedures, Safety, and New Developments*, pp 193–205, Zatuchni GI, Sciarra JJ and Speidel JJ (eds)  Harper & Row, Hagerstown, MD, 1979
12  Barr MM  Midtrimester abortions — 12 to 20 weeks by dilatation and evacuation method under local anesthesia  *Adv Plann Parent* 13  16–20, 1978
13  Berry FN and Peterson WF  D&E plus suction in midtrimester abortion  *The Female Patient* pp 86–88, 1978
14  Boyd C  Unpublished data
15  Burnhill MS  Vaginal second-trimester abortion  In  *Risks, Benefits and Controversies in Fertility Control* Sciarra JJ, Speidel JJ and Zatuchni G (eds) pp 331–347  Harper & Row, Hagerstown, 1978
16  DeLee ST  Termination of pregnancy in the midtrimester using a new technique  Preliminary report  *Int Surg* 61  545–546, 1976
17  Glick E and Sacks M  Public health aspects of dilatation and evacuation  Presented at the 106th Annual Meeting of the American Public Health Association, Los Angeles, CA, October 14, 1978
18  Goodman MP  Vacuum dilatation and evacuation for midtrimester abortion  *J Reprod Med* (in press)
19  Grimes DA, Hulka JF and McCutchen ME  Midtrimester abortion by dilatation and evacuation versus intra-amniotic instillation of prostaglandin F2a  a randomized clinical trial  *Am J Obstet Gynecol* 137  785–790, 1980
20  Hanson MS  D&E midtrimester abortion  Presented at 16th Annual Meeting, Association of Planned Parenthood Physicians, San Diego, CA, October 25–27, 1977
21  Hern WM and Oakes AG  Multiple laminaria treatment in early midtrimester outpatient suction abortion  a preliminary report  *Adv Plann Parent* 12  93–97, 1977
22  Hodari AA, Peralta J, Quiroga PJ and Gerbi EB  Dilatation and curettage for second

trimester abortions *Am J Obstet Gynecol* 127 850–854, 1977

23 Hubacker AS D&E for late second trimester abortion *Adv Plann Parent* 15 119–122, 1981

24 Kaltreider NB, Goldsmith S and Margolis AJ The impact of midtrimester abortion techniques on patients and staff *Am J Obstet Gynecol* 135 235–238, 1979

25 Kophk L Early midtrimester abortion by curettage Presented at 13th Annual Meeting, Association of Planned Parenthood Physicians, Los Angeles, CA, April 7, 1975

26 Livingston RM Affidavit to the Superior Court of the New Jersey Appellate Division — Bergen County, October 21, 1977

27 Meadowbrook Women's Clinic D&E procedures *Meadowbrook Memo* 3 (1) 1, 1978

28 Stubblefield PG, Albrecht BH, Koos B, et al A randomized study of 12 mm and 15 9 mm cannulas in midtrimester abortion by laminaria and vacuum curettage *Fertil Steril* 29 512–517, 1978

29 Tietze C and Lewit S Joint Program for the Study of Abortion (JPSA) early medical complications of legal abortion *Stud Fam Plann* 3 97–124, 1972

30 Tietze C and Lewit S Early medical complications of abortion by saline Joint Program for the Study of Abortion (JPSA) *Stud Fann Plann* 4 133–138, 1973

31 Stewart GK and Goldstein P Medical and surgical complications of therapeutic abortions *Obstet Gynecol* 40 539–542, 1972

32 Brenner WE and Edelman DA Dilatation and evacuation at 13 to 15 weeks gestation versus intra-amniotic saline after 15 weeks gestation *Contraception* 10 171–180, 1974

33 Grimes DA, Schulz KF, Cates W Jr and Tyler CW Jr Midtrimester abortion by dilatation and evacuation A safe and practical alternative *N Engl J Med* 296 1141–1145, 1977

34 Goldsmith S, Kaltreider NB and Margolis AJ Second trimester abortion by dilatation and evacuation (D&E) surgical technique and psychological reactions Presented at the 15th Annual Meeting, Association of Planned Parenthood Physicians, Atlanta, GA, October 13, 1977

35 Smith RG, Steinhoff PG and Palmore JA Potential reduction of medical complications from induced abortions *Int Gynaecol Obstet* 15 337–346, 1978

36 Manabe Y Artificial abortion at midpregnancy by mechanical stimulation of the uterus *Am J Obstet Gynecol* 105 132–146, 1969

37 Manabe Y and Nakajima A Laminaria-metreurynter method of midterm abortion in Japan *Obstet Gynecol* 40 612–615, 1972

38 Manabe Y Metreurynter-induced abortions at midpregnancy *Am J Obstet Gynecol* 99 557–561, 1967

39 Manabe Y, Nakajima A and Griggs JF Uterine contractility and placental histology in abortion by laminaria and metreurynter *Obstet Gynecol* 41 753–759, 1973

40 Nishimura T and Manabe Y Oxytocin sensitivity and effects of estrogen and progesterone on metreurynter-induced abortions at midpregnancy *Am J Obstet Gynecol* 98 1087–1090, 1967

41 Burnett LS, Wentz AC and King TM Techniques of pregnancy termination Part II *Obstet Gynecol Surv* 29 6–42, 1974

42 Grimes DA, Cates W Jr and Tyler CW Jr Death after legal abortion by catheter placement *Am J Obstet Gynecol* 127 219–222, 1977

43 Mullick B, Brenner WE and Berger GS Termination of pregnancy with intrauterine devices *Am J Obstet Gynecol* 116 305–308, 1973

44 Berger GS, Bourne JP, Tyler CW Jr, et al Termination of pregnancy by 'super coils' Morbidity associated with a new method of second trimester abortion *Am J Obstet Gynecol* 116 297–304, 1973

45 Grimes DA, Cates W Jr and Selik RM Fatal septic abortion in the United States, 1975–1977 Obstet Gynecol 57 739–744, 1981

46 Niswander KR, Klein M and Randall CL Therapeutic abortion indications and techniques *Obstet Gynecol* 28 124–129, 1966

# 8. INTRA-AMNIOTIC HYPERTONIC SALINE INSTILLATION IN THE SECOND TRIMESTER

## THOMAS D. KERENYI

Hypertonic saline induction of late abortion after more than a decade of experience, including modification and/or combination with new abortifacients, has remained the most reliable and safest of methods to date. This physician's personal experience of over 12 000 cases invites the conclusion that saline induction, provided the procedure is properly executed, is a safe and effective technique. Currently, it is still the most widely used method of terminating late second trimester pregnancies [1].

The history of hypertonic saline instillation is relatively recent; it only became widely used in the United States and Western Europe in the 1960s. Its post-war acceptance was impeded by the high rates of complications and mortality reported from Japan [2], attributable to improper utilization of the technique, and infusions performed by inexperienced practitioners in inadequate facilities on patients who were not screened for pre-existing medical disorders. However, indiscriminate and injudicious use of the technique only temporarily halted its eventual usage.

The technique's emergence in the United States in the 1960s [3, 4] began as an alternative technique to surgical procedures, i.e., hysterotomy. It evolved to become a technique almost exclusively performed by transabdominal instillation of the solution directly into the amniotic sac. However, a transvaginal approach is also feasible [5].

The exact mechanism of action by which hypertonic saline induces abortion is still under debate. Several theories have been proposed: 1) a suspension of the 'placental defense mechanism' which thereby depresses progesterone production [6–11]; 2) prostaglandins generated locally resulting in uterine contractions and expulsion of the fetus [12, 13]; 3) acute salt poisoning of the products of conception resulting in fetal death and onset of uterine activity [14, 15]; 4) oxytocin release from the posterior pituitary which, in turn, stimulates myometrial contractility [16].

It is doubtful that the oxytocin theory is operational and that acute salt poisoning is a primary pathway. However, both the decline in the progesterone block and the generation of prostaglandins probably play an important role in the initiation and/or acceleration of myometrial contractility. The two combined probably constitute the final pathway to all endogenous or exogenous uterine stimulation. This comprehensive theory, advanced by

M.J.N.C. Keirse et al. (eds.), Second Trimester Pregnancy Termination. All rights reserved.
Copyright © 1982 Martinus Nijhoff Publishers, The Hague/Boston/London.

Csapo, accommodates the hypothesis both for spontaneous and induced uterine activity at any stage of pregnancy and is known as the 'see-saw' theory [11].

Final agreement also has not been reached on the desirability of full hospitalization. Since it is a two-stage procedure, it is tempting to perform the first part in an ambulatory setting and then expect the patient to return for the active phase of labor and expulsion [17, 18]. The desirability of such an approach is a uniquely North American problem where the cost of hospitalization is so prohibitive that the choice of procedure is almost dictated by 'cost-effectiveness' rather than what is the safest; thus, in most cases, the procedure of choice becomes the one that requires only over-night hospitalization. Had it not been for this pressure to compress the instillation-abortion time (I.A.T.) to under 24 hours, the combination procedures such as hypertonic saline and prostaglandin, hypertonic urea and prostaglandin, and oxytocin augmentation might not have come into existence even though the margin of safety is narrower than with hypertonic saline alone. Because of the increased rate of complications, despite a shorter time interval achieved, it is now required in most states that the patient be hospitalized in a fully equipped and well-staffed facility throughout the procedure [19].

Careful screening of the patient for pre-existing medical conditions is strongly advised. While they may not represent contraindication, their appropriate handling is important. Conditions such as sickle-cell anemia, cardiac or renal disease, etc. should be recognized and evaluated prior to carrying out the procedure [19–21].

TECHNIQUE

The transabdominal instillation is performed in the supine position and the transvaginal instillation in the lithotomy position. The patient's bladder is emptied prior to the procedure; then the lower abdomen is cleansed with an antiseptic solution and draped with sterile towels. Local anesthetic is used to infiltrate the instillation site. It is best selected by prior sonographic scanning of the uterus to: 1) determine the accurate gestational age and 2) select the optimum site where the amniotic fluid pool is best approached. Then a needle with an obturator is inserted into the uterus. Some adjustment of the needle's depth or angle may be required before fluid freely issues from it. To verify that it is indeed amniotic fluid and not maternal urine, an indicator strip is used to test for the presence of protein and alkalinity, charateristic of amniotic fluid.

Not only is it important to establish a free-flow but a significant amount of fluid should also be removed (100 to 400 ml). Instillation without any amniotic fluid removal may not result in too rapid an increase of intra-amniotic pressure resulting in early rupture of membranes with attendant sequelae, but also in overdilution of the instilled hypertonic solution thereby causing missed labor or live abortion [8]. The optimum amount of saline instilled is $\pm 200$ ml (with a range of 150–250 ml) depending on the size of the gestation. The volume and concentration relationships crucial to successful procedure are discussed elsewhere [8]. In an effort to minimize needle displacement during the instillation procedure, some practitioners recommend use of catheters placed through a large-bore needle [21, 22]. In the author's experience, a $3\frac{1}{2}$ inch long disposable 18 gauge spinal needle provides the best 'feel'. It minimizes obstruction, leakage and, last but not least, early recognition of saline reaction. The 18 gauge needle allows the deposition of the hypertonic solution by gravity technique (by drip-infusion from an intravenous closed system set-up) in approximately ten minutes. If by accident the needle is malpositioned, e.g., if it is not in the amniotic sac, the rapidly-appearing side-effects allow the operator to shut-off the infusion before the adverse reaction becomes too severe or irreversible [23]. If the cavity is lost or if the tap is bloody, infusion of isotonic (0.9% NaCl) solution is quite helpful after adjustment of the needle's position to verify proper intra-amniotic placement.

EFFECTIVENESS

The instillation-abortion time (I.A.T.) in unstimulated patients is approximately 36 hours. Depending on the concentration of the stimulant (intravenous oxytocin), the I.A.T. may be pushed down to under 24 hours. However, experience has shown that over-stimulation may lead to a significant increase in the rate of complications, particularly cervical tears and hemorrhage. If the patient is left unstimulated, the fetus is expelled within 72 hours in approximately 97% of the patients [24]. Even in Pitocin augmented cases, a second amniotic infusion with hypertonic saline may become necessary in 1% of the cases after 48 hours because of failure of expulsion. If the time factor is crucial and if there is no evidence of uterine activity within 24 hours, a second instillation may be contemplated. The concentration of hypertonic solution is significantly decreased with 24 hours [8] and the dangers resulting from a second instillation are probably negligible. However, if significant cervical dilatation and effacement has already taken place, an amniotomy is preferred to reinfusion and frequently results in acceleration of the labor process. Total absence of labor should alert the operator to the possibility of ovarian cyst infusion which must be ruled out [23].

In patients for whom the instillation could not be completed, it is mandatory to check for the presence or absence of fetal heart sounds. Due to accidental needle removal or minor saline reaction, the administered amount of hypertonic saline may not have been adequate and thus not feticidal. Live abortion may be encountered, one of the emotionally and prognostically most disturbing complications. In the author's opinion, it will not occur unless misjudgment of the gestational stage or incomplete infusion are carried out. The result is either overdilution or insufficient hypertonicity, amounting to the same: lack of feticidal effect.

MORBIDITY

The method, in experienced hands, has proved to be safe. However, even in experienced hands, several medical complications have been recognized to appear in less than 5% of the cases. These are hypernatremia (greater than 160 mEq/l serum sodium), coagulopathy (varying degree of blood coagulation disorder), hemorrhage (greater than 500 ml blood loss), and infection and/or fever.

Mild hypernatremia can be recognized (1 per 200 cases) when the patient complains of facial flushing, restlessness, thirst, headache, or if there is evidence of hypertension, or bradycardia or apnea is noted [21, 23]. It is almost invariably the result of inadvertent injection of the hypertonic saline into the patient's vascular system rather than into the amniotic sac. The patient's clear sensorium is of utmost importance in recognizing these early signs. In a heavily sedated patient, the full load of hypertonic solution delivered in the wrong compartment may result in irreversible damage to the central nervous system which would manifest in seizures or coma. Yet, it should be completely avoidable by the use of proper technique [23]. Should it still occur, it may be life-threatening [25, 26]. As soon as it is suspected, hypernatremia should be treated with intravenous infusion of normal saline, 5% dextrose solution or the oral administration of fluids in the milder cases. Subsequent urinary output and vital signs should be carefully monitored.

Several factors which participate in the coagulability of blood change significantly 6–12 hours after instillation of hypertonic saline. Almost all parameters return to normal in 24 hours and severe clotting disorders are rare [23, 26, 27].

Cohen and Ballard [26] found only ten cases of clinically serious coagulopathy in the review of almost 5000 cases over a six-year period, induced by hypertonic saline. In the author's experience, the incidence of clinically recognizable coagulopathy was 0.3%. Early oxytocin administration increases the risk of coagulopathy. If the patient develops clotting disorder, fresh blood or cryoprecipitate should be rapidly transfused and the uterus should be examined to insure that all products of conception have been evacuated.

The most frequent complications following hypertonic saline instillation are hemorrhage and infection. Berger and Kerenyi [24] in over 4000 patients reported an overall incidence of 5.5%. Hemorrhage increased with prolonged retention of the placenta [25–27] and the author recommends the removal of the placenta when feasible within 2–4 hours unless significant bleeding requires it earlier. In various studies the reported incidence of transfusion varied from 5 to 7% [26].

Fever related to infection has been reported to be 2.2–6.2% of cases [26]. Risk of infection has been shown to increase when the I.A.T. exceeds 48 hours [25–27]. This notion has led to the almost universal use of augmenting agents such as oxytocin [28]. However, their use does not have to precede the onset of spontaneous contractions or exceed the usual physiologic dosages. Prevention of infection is, naturally, best maintained through strict adherence to high standards of sterile technique. However, once infection is recognized and is suspected to be bacterial in nature, intravenous antibiotics are the method of choice. Persistent infections must be precisely diagnosed by utilization of cultures and appropriate sensitivity studies. It is also mandatory to establish that retained products of conception with nidation of infection are not the cause for lack of response.

Cervical tears or other uterine injuries are seldom associated with intra-amniotic instillation alone. Augmentation either by high doses of intravenous oxytocin or prostaglandins by various routes are more likely to be the actual culprits [29, 30]. Cervical tears may be repaired transvaginally or may necessitate laparotomy, depending on the location and the extent of the injury.

Water intoxication may be prevented by using no electrolyte-free solutions for intravenous infusion during hypertonic saline instillation. In addition, when Pitocin is used, no more than 40 mU/min (2 ampules = 20 International Units per 100 ml over 8 hours) should be utilized. When oxytocin is added to electrolyte-containing solution, even with high doses (5–10 ampules per liter), water intoxication does not occur [8, 9, 23].

Live abortions, as previously discussed, are extremely rare and usually are associated with breach of the standard protocol. Therefore, it is strongly recommended that if any difficulty is encountered during the instillation, the fetal heart should be checked 2 hours after instillation. If still present, appropriate measures should be taken as discussed above. It is again emphasized that the most frequent source of error leading to overdilution and lack of feticidal effect is the misjudgment of the patient's gestational age. It is the author's observation that even the most experienced clinicians are frequently mistaken about size estimation in the midtrimester of pregnancy by as much as ± 2 weeks and occasionally by as much as ± 4 weeks. When ultrasound cephalometry is employed, the upper limit of 24 weeks gestation (menstrual age) should be 60 to 63 mm of the fetal biparital diameter utilizing an outer-to-outer table measurement [31].

MORTALITY

Schiffer [31] has reviewed the main factors leading to maternal death and found that they are: complications secondary to incomplete abortion with hemorrhage and sepsis, complications which arise from the use of other agents in attempts to abbreviate the I.A.T. and complications secondary to pre-existing medical conditions which are not compatible with this method of abortion. According to the 1977 data reported by Tyler of the United States Center for Disease Control, only six deaths were associated with late abortions, a decrease from eighteen in 1973, resulting in a mortality rate of 6.5 per 100 000 procedures [32].

Even though these statistics may show a significant potential morbidity and mortality, one must consider what the alternatives are to those patients who have advanced to the late second trimester without either recognizing that they were pregnant, or for various medical, social, or psychological reasons have decided to abort their pregnancies. If these patients go to term rather than abort the pregnancy late, they show a proportionately higher rate of complications than the overall population as well as a predictably more dismal future for their offspring [33, 34].

SUMMARY

It is of paramount importance to recognize that regardless of what hypertonic solution (saline, urea, glucose, etc.) is instilled into the amniotic sac, the resultant basic process is the induction of labor. Whether this event takes place at the end of the second or the end of the third trimester it is dependent upon the active participation of the myometrium in the process of self-evacuation. In case of mishaps, the greater the uterine size the more severe are the ensuing complications. Associated with the most frequent obstetrical complications such as hemorrhage or infection, this is particularly applicable. The time-perfected 'expectant mangement' employed on labor floors represents the most appropriate set-up for these late abortions induced by hypertonic instillations. Such an approach includes the continuous presence of obstetrically trained personnel, nurses of physicians, supervised by experts. A woman in labor, whether the onset was spontaneous or induced and whether at 5 or at 9 months of gestation, in the author's opinion, deserves nothing less than that.

86

REFERENCES

1 American College of Obstetricians and Gynecologists Methods of Midtrimester Abortion *Techn Bull*, 56 1979
2 Wagatsuma T Intra-amniotic injection of saline for therapeutic abortion *Am J Obstet Gynecol* 93 743–745, 1965
3 Kerenyi TD, Jaffin H and Wood EC Termination of missed abortion and the induction of labor in midtrimester pregnancy *Am J Obstet Gynecol* 84 602–608, 1962
4 Csapo AI Termination of pregnancy by the intra-amniotic injection of hypertonic saline In *The Yearbook of Obstetrics and Gynecology, 1966–1976* Greenhill JP (ed), pp 126–163 Yearbook Medical, Chicago, 1966
5 Ruttner BT Termination of midtrimester pregnancy by transvaginal intra-amniotic injection of hypertonic solution *Obstet Gynecol* 28 601–605, 1966
6 Bengtsson L and Csapo AI Oxytocin response withdrawal, and reinforcement of denfense mechanism of the human uterus at midpregnancy *Am J Obstet Gynecol* 83 1083'1093, 1962
7 Csapo AI, Knobil E, Pulkkinen M, Van Der Molen HJ, Sommerville IF and Wiest WG Progesterone withdrawal during hypertonic saline-induced abortions *Am J Obstet Gynecol* 105 1132–1134, 1969
8 Kerenyi TD and Muzsnai D Volume and sodium concentration studies in 300 saline-induced abortions *Am J Obstet Gynecol* 121 590–596, 1975
9 Kerenyi TD Midtrimester abortion In *The Abortion Experience*, pp 383–399 Osofsky HJ and Osofsky JD (eds), Harper & Row, Hagertown, 1973
10 Tyack AJ, Parsons RJ, Millar DR, Pennington G and Hall R Plasma progesterone changes in abortion induced by hypertonic saline in the second trimester of pregnancy *J Obstet Gynaecol Br Commonw* 80 518–552, 1973
11 Csapo AI The 'see-saw' theory of the regulatory mechanism of pregnancy *Am J Obstet Gynecol* 121 578, 1975
12 Gustavii B The distribution within the placenta, myometrium, and decidua of $^{24}$Na-labelled hypertonic saline solution following intra-amniotic or extra-amniotic injection *Br J Obstet Gynaecol* 82 734–739, 1975
13 Honore LH The mechanism of midtrimester abortion induced by intra-amniotic instillation of hypertonic saline a modification of Gustavii's lysosomal hypothesis *Am J Obstet Gynecol* 126 1011, 1976
14 Galen RS, Chauhan P, Wietzner H and Navarro C Fetal pathology and mechanism of fetal death in saline-induced abortion a study of 143 gestations and critical review of the literature *Am J Obstet gynecol* 120 347–355, 1974
15 Myers RE, Symchych P, Strauss L, Comas A, Figueroa-Longo J, Kerenyi T and Adamsons K Morphologic changes of uterine wall following intra-amniotic injection of hypertonic saline in the rhesus monkey *Am J Obstet Gynecol* 119 877–888, 1974
16 Short RV, Wagner G, Fuchs AR and Fuchs F Progesterone concentrations in uterine venous blood after intra-amniotic injection of hypertonic saline in midpregnancy *Am J Obstet Gynecol* 91 132–136, 1965
17 Kerenyi TD Outpatient intra-amniotic injection of hypertonic saline *Clin Obstet gynecol* 15 124–140, 1971
18 Tietze C and Lewit S Highlights of the Joint Program for the Study of Abortion (JPSA) early medical complications of legal abortion In *Advances in Planne Parenthood*, Lewit S (ed), Vol 8, pp 173–176 Excerpta Medica, Amsterdam, 1973
19 Zuspan FP, Ballard CA, Bieniarz J, Brenner WE, Corson SL, Kaiser IH, Kerenyi TD, King TM and Tietze C Second trimester abortion — a symposium by correspondence *J Reprod Med* 16 47–64, 1976
20 Kerenyi TD Technique of late abortion In *Abortion Techniques and Services*, Lewit S (ed), pp 17–22 Proceedings of the Conference, New York, June 3–5, 1971 Excerpta Medica, Amsterdam, 1972
21 Perry G, Schulman H and Wong TC Modified saline abortion for medically high-risk patients *Obstet Gynecol* 44 571–578, 1974

22  Kerenyi TD, Mandelman N and Sherman DH  Five thousand consecutive saline inductions  *Am J Obstet Gynecol* 116  593–600, 1973

23  Schulman H, Kaiser IH and Randolph G  Outpatient saline abortion  *Obstet Gynecol* 37  521–526, 1971

24  Berger GS and Kerenyi TD  Control of morbidity associated with saline abortion  *Adv Plann Parenthood* 9  31–37, 1975

25  Burnett LS, Wentz AC and King TM  Techniques of pregnancy termination Part 2  *Obstet Gynecol Survey* 29  7–42, 1974

26  Cohen E and Ballard CA  Consumptive coagulopathy associated with intra-amniotic saline instillation and the effect of intravenous oxytocin  *Obstet gynecol* 43  300–303, 1974

27  Lauersen NH and Schulman JD  Oxytocin administration in midtrimester saline abortions  *Am J Obstet Gynecol* 115  420–430, 1973

28  Horowitz DA  Uterine rupture following attempted saline abortion with oxytocin in a grandmultiparous patient  *Obstet Gynecol* 43  921–922, 1974

29  Hirsch JS  Cervical fistula as a complication of midtrimester abortion  *Obstet Gynecol* 41  478, 1973

30  Lauersen HH and Birnbaum SJ  Water intoxication associated with oxytocin administration during saline-induced abortion  *Am J Obstet Gynecol* 121  2–6, 1975

31  Schiffer MA, Pakter J and Clahr J  Mortality associated with hypertonic saline abortion  *Obstet Gynecol* 42  759–764, 1973

32  United States Center for Disease Control (CDC)  *Abortion surveillance – Annual Summary 1977* (HEW Publication No (CDC) 1979) Atlanta, GA 1979

33  Rovinsky JJ  Impact of permissive abortion statute on community health care  *Obstet Gynecol* 41  781–788, 1973

34  Brenner WE  Second trimester interruption of pregnancy  *Progress in Gynecology*, Vol 6, In Taymor ML and Green TH (eds), Grune & Stratton, New York, 1975

# 9. EXTRA-AMNIOTIC ETHACRIDINE (RIVANOL®)*-CATHETER TECHNIQUE FOR MIDTRIMESTER ABORTION

CARL-AXEL INGEMANSON

Since the early 1960s the most frequently used method for second trimester abortion in Sweden has been the intra- or extra-amniotic instillation of hypertonic saline. Reports of three deaths and a number of serious complications in 6161 saline abortions in Sweden [1] prompted investigation of other methods.

Japan is undoubtedly the country with the greatest experience of legal abortions. Hypertonic saline was used extensively in Japan at the end of the 1940s to induce abortion in midtrimester pregnancies, but after Hashizume [2] and others reported a high frequency of serious complications — including 13 deaths in 6611 abortion cases — other methods have been preferred. One of the most frequently used methods for midtrimester abortion in Japan over the last 25 years is the extra-amniotic instillation of 30–200 ml of an 0.1% solution of Rivanol in combination with the insertion of a rubber catheter into the uterus.

## RIVANOL

Rivanol (6,9-diamino-2-oxyethyl acridine lactate) is a yellow dye with strong antiseptic properties. As a medicament this acridine derivative has been useful as an antiseptic agent for wounds and for infections of the genito-urinary tract and nasopharynx, and has been used in 0.04–0.05% solution. In the pre-antibiotic era moderate amounts of 0.1% Rivanol were used intravenously in man in Japan without any signs of toxic effects.

Large volumes, however, of an 0.1% Rivanol solution can be nephrotoxic. Pytel et al. (3) in the Soviet Union reported five cases of acute renal insufficiency, four of which were of a temporary nature, with the use of 500–700 ml 0.1% Rivanol in late legal abortion. In our experience, we have one case with temporary anuria after having 140 ml of an incorrectly prepared 1.0% Rivanol solution instilled extra-amniotically [4]. Follow-up studies 2 months after the episode showed completely normal renal function. Thus it is important to consider that any solution deposited in the uterus can be absorbed

---

* Registered trademark, Farbwerke Hoechst AG, Frankfurt, West Germany.

rapidly into the systematic circulation. For this reason the solution chosen for intra-uterine infusion should be as safe to the woman as if the same amount of solution were injected intravenously.

The antiseptic nature of the solution is also an important factor. Many septic complications have been reported using distilled water, hypertonic saline and glucose solutions of varied concentrations. Thus moderate amounts of a 0.1% solution of Rivanol can be used as it is safe to the patient and antiseptic. 30–200 ml of 0.1% Rivanol solution has been used extensively in Japan over the last 25 years and neither death nor any other serious complication has been reported to date with these amounts.

Studies by Gustavii [5] suggest that the abortifacient effect of the Rivanol-catheter method is due to prostaglandin synthesis in the decidual cells. This concept is supported by studies by Ölund [6], who has shown that indomethacin, a strong prostaglandin synthetase inhibitor, significantly prolongs the induction-abortion interval in patients undergoing midtrimester abortion by extra-amniotic Rivanol-catheter.

### EXPERIENCE WITH THE RIVANOL-CATHETER METHOD

In a pilot study comprising 106 consecutive cases of legal abortion in the 13th to 20th week of gestation the author compared 20% extra-amniotic saline and the extra-amniotic Rivanol-catheter method [4]. Alternating patients were administered either 20% saline extra-amniotically or 0.1% Rivanol extra-amniotically plus catheter insertion into the uterus. The amount of solution used was in both groups 10 ml per week of pregnancy up to a maximum of 150 ml. In both groups a catheter was inserted approximately 4 cm past the internal os and after an aspiration check for blood 20% saline or 0.1% Rivanol was gently instilled extra-amniotically for 3–5 min, 10 ml per week of pregnancy up to a maximum of 150 ml. In the saline cases the catheter was withdrawn immediately after instillation was completed, but in the Rivanol cases the catheter, a rubber catheter Nelaton no. 16, was inserted farther up into the cavity until only 1 or 2 cm protruded from the cervix. No oxytocin was used in this study. The catheter was left in place until abortion occurred.

No serious complications occurred, but there was a considerable difference in side effects between the two groups (Table 1). In the saline group 12 patients experienced considerable pain and 4 slight pain during instillation; 4 experienced nausea and vomiting, 3 a sudden temporary fall in blood pressure and 4 a sensation of overall warmth. Side effects in the Rivanol-catheter group were limited to one case of slight pain during instillation. Signs of infection were more common in the saline group. Sixteen patients had a temperature rise to more than 38° C compared with 5 in the Rivanol group.

*Table 1* Comparison of extraamniotic saline with Rivanol for abortion at 13 to 20 weeks of gestation [4]

| Side effect or complication | 20% NaCl n = 53 | Rivanol + catheter n = 53 |
|---|---|---|
| Slight pain during instillation | 4 | 1 |
| Considerable pain during instillation | 12 | 0 |
| Nausea and vomiting | 4 | 0 |
| Fall in blood pressure to < 100 mg Hg | 3 | 0 |
| Feeling of overall warmth | 4 | 0 |
| Temperature rise of 38° C during hospitalization | 16 | 5 |
| No of above with > 38° C for 48 hours or more | 7 | 2 |

The fever lasted usually only one day but 7 patients in the saline group and 2 in the Rivanol group were in fever for 2 days or more. The abortion rate was higher at 48 and 72 hours in the Rivanol catheter group but the difference was not significant.

Svanberg and Himmelman [7] studied 302 consecutive cases of extra-amniotic saline abortions and 200 consecutive cases of extra-amniotic Rivanol-catheter abortions. The catheter technique was different from our technique. A no. 16 Foley catheter with 10 cm$^3$ balloon was used and left in place for 24 hours. If contractions had not started within 24 hours an intravenous infusion of oxytocin was given [8]. The frequency of infection and bleeding was significantly higher in the saline group (Table 2). In the Rivanol group there was manifest infection in 1%, suspected infection in 8%, and bleeding in 1.5%; in the saline group manifest infection occurred in 6%, suspected infection in 20%, and bleeding in 6%.

Himmelman et al. [8] compared extra-amniotic Rivanol catheter and extra-amniotic prostaglandin $F_{2\alpha}$ ($PGF_{2\alpha}$) with respect to time factors and complications in second trimester abortions. The complications in the $PGF_{2\alpha}$ group were significantly higher than in the Rivanol group, and manifest infection and bleeding were each significantly more frequent in the $PGF_{2\alpha}$ group (Table 2).

*Table 2* Complication rates with different abortion methods in the second trimester (from Himmelman et al [8])

| Extra-amniotic administration of | No of cases | Type of complication (%) | | | |
|---|---|---|---|---|---|
| | | Bleeding | Manifest infection | Suspected infection | Total |
| Rivanol | 200 | 1 5 | 1 | 8 | 10 5 |
| $PGF_{2\alpha}$ | 50 | 8 | 8 | 6 | 22 |
| Hypertonic saline | 302 | 6 | 6 | 20 | 29 |

SAFETY AND SUCCESS RATE

Data collected from eight gynaecological departments in Sweden on 2058 consecutive Rivanol midtrimester abortions did not show any fatal or life-threatening complications. The only major complications encountered were one case of cervical fistula in a 16 year old nullipara with a rigid cervix and one case of cervical laceration. I believe we can state that the extra-amniotic Rivanol-catheter method is a safe procedure when moderate doses of 0.1% Rivanol are given. The complication rate is very low and compares favourably with other methods of second trimester abortion.

Another requirement of a good method of second trimester abortion is a high success rate within a reasonable period of time. The Rivanol method has a high success rate within 48–72 hours of instillation. In different studies the abortion rate within 24 hours is 28–52%, within 48 hours 79–100% and within 72 hours 88–100% (Table 3).

The abortion rate is influenced by the gestational week but neither age nor parity affect the results. The abortion rate is significantly lower in the 13th and 14th week of pregnancy than in later gestational weeks [8]. In studies comparing Rivanol-catheter and extra-amniotic $PGF_{2\alpha}$ there is a higher abortion rate at 24 hours with prostaglandin, but at 48 hours there is no statistically significant difference [8, 9]. In the Rivanol-catheter study with the best results [9] — 100% abortion within 48 hours — a Foley catheter with a large 30 $cm^3$ balloon was used. Fylling and Refsdal [10] tested different catheter techniques and obtained the fastest induction-abortion intervals when using a Foley catheter.

At present, one of the most popular methods in Japan for late legal abortion is the use of laminaria tents in the cervical canal followed by a metre-urynter in the lower uterine cavity to give a mechanical stretch (Manabe, personal communication, 1980). By using a Foley catheter with a big balloon

Table 3. The extra-amniotic Rivanol-catheter method for termination of pregnancy.

| Authors | No. of cases | Amount of 0.1% Rivanol | Oxytocin given | Abortion within 24 h (%) | Abortion within 48 h (%) | Abortion within 72 h (%) |
|---|---|---|---|---|---|---|
| Ingemanson [4] | 182 | 50–150 | no | 28 | 79 | 92 |
| Svanberg and Himmelman [7] | 200 | 130–150 | yes | 29 | 77 | 88 |
| Fylling and Refsdal[10] | 69 | 100–200 | yes | 36 | 78 | 88 |
| Ölund and Larsson [9] | 23 | 130–150 | yes | ? | 100 | 100 |
| Butler [12] | 44 | 50 | yes | 52 | 92 | 94 |

in the Rivanol-catheter induced abortions, one will most likely create a metreurynter effect and thereby speed up the abortion process. Thus we have reason to believe that our present Rivanol-catheter technique gives optimal results.

TECHNIQUE:

1. Thorough cleansing of the vagina with an antiseptic solution (0.05% Chlorhexidine).
2. A Foley catheter no. 18–20 with a 30 cm$^3$ balloon, filled with 0.1% Rivanol is introduced via the cervical canal just past the internal os.
3. The catheter balloon is filled with 30 ml physiological saline.
4. Aspiration check for blood.
5. If no blood flows into the syringe, 150 ml (irrespective of the week of pregnancy) of a 0.1% solution of Rivanol is gently instilled in the extra-ovular space in 3–4 minutes.
6. The catheter is fixed to the thigh with a slight stretch to prevent leakage and to cause a metreurynter effect.
7. The catheter is left in place for 24 hours (if the patient is not aborting earlier).
8. If the abortion has not started the following morning an intravenous infusion of oxytocin (70 IU in 1000 ml 5.5% glucose) is started and this infusion is repeated every 12th hour until abortion occurs.
9. If no abortion has occurred within 48 hours the above procedure is repeated.

The Rivanol-catheter method can be combined with prostaglandin administration. Martin et al. [11] and Ölund and Larsson [9] gave extra-amniotic PGF$_{2\alpha}$ after the instillation of Rivanol. This modification combines the immediate uterotonic effect of prostaglandin with the delayed response to Rivanol, and it is possible to obtain a higher abortion rate within 24 hours than with Rivanol-catheter alone.

CONCLUSION

In summary, the extra-amniotic Rivanol-catheter method offers many advantages in second trimester abortion. It is safe to the patient even in the hands of less experienced doctors in the recommended concentrations and doses. It is an easy, usually painless, once-only procedure. The complication rate is low. There is a high success rate within 48 hours and the abortion process can be accelerated with additional prostaglandin. The method is inexpensive and has no known contraindications. The only disadvantage is that the method does not generally cause foetal death and it is therefore not recommended to exceed the 20th week of pregnancy.

REFERENCES

1. Bengtsson LP: Legal abortion by intrauterine injections. *Läkartidningen* 64: 5037–5053, 1967.
2. Hashizume K: *Jap Obstet Gynecol Soc* 2: 145–000, 1950.
3. Pytel AY, Lopatkin NA and Kuchinsky IN: Acute Renal insufficiency associated with intrauterine retromembranous administration of Rivanol for the interruption of pregnancy and its treatment with hemodialysis. *Akush Ginekol (Mosk)* 39: 5–00, 1963.
4. Ingemanson CA:Legal abortion by extraamniotic instillation of Rivanol in combination with rubber catheter insertion into the uterus after the twelfth week of pregnancy. *Am J Obstet Gynecol* 115: 211–215, 1973.
5. Gustavii G: Rivanol induced alterations of cultured cells. *Contraception* 1: 89–00, 1977.
6. Ölund A: The effect of indomethacin on the instillation-abortion interval in Rivanol-induced midtrimester abortion. *Acta Obstet Gynecol Scand* 58: 121–122, 1979.
7. Svanberg SG and Himmelman A: Late abortion by the Rivanol-catheter method. *Nya forskningar och rön* 7: 269–277, 1972.
8. Himmelman A, Myhrman P and Svanberg SG: Induction of second trimester abortion. Comparison between Rivanol and prostaglandin $F_2$ regarding time factors and complications. *Contraception* 12: 645–654, 1975.
9. Ölund A and Larsson B: Comparison of extraamniotic instillation of Rivanol and $PFG_2$ either separately or in combination followed by oxytocin for second trimester abortion. *Acta Obstet Gynecol Scand* 57: 333–336, 1978.
10. Fylling P and Refsdal A: Rivanol-induced midtrimester abortion. *Arch Gynäkol* 215: 359–363, 1973.
11. Martin JN, Bygdeman M, Leader A and Wiqvist N: Early second trimester abortion by the extraamniotic instillation of Rivanol solution and a single $PGF_{2\alpha}$ dose. Contraception 11: 523–531, 1975.
12. Butler JC: Ethacridine-catheter method in second trimester abortion. In: *Pregnancy Termination*, Zatuchni GI, Sciarra JJ and Speidel JJ (eds), pp. 277–281. Harper & Row, Hagerstown, MD, 1979.

## 10. FACT AND FANCY IN THE TERMINATION OF MOLAR PREGNANCY WITH PARTICULAR REFERENCE TO UTERINE STIMULANTS

MARC J.N.C. KEIRSE

Since molar pregnancy predisposes to severe haemorrhage, pre-eclampsia and the development of choriocarcinoma, evacuation of the uterine contents as soon as possible is an essential part of its management. Theoretically, the termination of molar pregnancy needs to be less dependent on gestational age and uterine size than is the case in other pregnancies. The absence of foetal parts and would-be viability greatly reduces both the emotional and technical difficulties, whereas increasing gestational age does not of necessity exclude the use of the same techniques that can be applied in early pregnancy. As compared to other terminations, techniques for the evacuation of molar pregnancy may therefore appear to be virtually independent of gestational age. However, this is not the unqualified truth for uterine size. In molar pregnancy, uterine size is a far more important criterion than gestational age. This is particularly so since the relation between uterine size and gestational age differs greatly from the pattern observed in other pregnancies.

When this is taken into account, the termination of a molar pregnancy resembles that of any other pregnancy in at least two respects. Firstly, vacuum aspiration is universally considered as the treatment of choice when uterine size is below 12 to 14 weeks. Secondly, a much larger uterus evokes a great deal of discussion on preferential methodology. In such discussions, it is not always easy to distinguish fact from fancy, and this applies to molar pregnancy too. The main purpose of this chapter is to enable us to differentiate between fact and fancy with regard to second trimester molar pregnancy. In this context, second trimester will remain rather undefined. On the one hand, it theoretically relates not to a gestational age but to a uterine size of 14 weeks or more. On the other hand, it may relate even more to uterine sizes beyond 16 weeks rather than 12 or 14 weeks, and may to some extent depend on the individual's experience with the evacuation of a rather large uterus. This ambiguity in defining second trimester molar pregnancy merely indicates that here too the trimester threshold should not be considered as a sharp dividing line but more as a continuum (Cates, chapter 5).

The discussion on preferential methods for the termination of molar pregnancy centres mainly on the merits and hazards of two approaches. Hysterotomy is no longer favoured and hysterectomy is only rarely indicated [1, 2]. Apart from a few proponents of alternative aids, such as laminaria tents, the primary choice is therefore mainly limited to vacuum aspiration, the use of oxytocic drugs or a combination of both. A consequence of this limitation of the methods of choice is that variables such as age, parity and the desire for further child bearing now have less influence on the selection of the mode of uterine evacuation.

Nevertheless, it remains difficult to gather enough insight in order to select the most appropriate approach in cases of second trimester molar pregnancy. This is not so surprising, when we consider the rarity of the condition on the one hand, and the fact that all of the currently favoured methods have been in use for less than a quarter of a century on the other hand. The use of high doses of oxytocin to stimulate the abortion of molar pregnancies was introduced in 1959 [3], but the use of vacuum aspiration and the administration of prostaglandins only date back to 1966 [4] and 1970 [5] respectively.

*Vacuum aspiration*

Since Brandes et al. [4] introduced vacuum aspiration of molar tissue irrespective of uterine size, the method has found many proponents. It is undoubtedly the method of choice when uterine size is below second trimester size or in the presence of spontaneous uterine contractility and a partially dilated cervix. Yet, in the presence of a firmly closed cervix and a large uterus, the risks may be greater than hitherto appreciated. Some authors [6] have encountered unexplained sudden deaths with such a procedure, but unfortunately no further details have appeared in the medical literature. A common pattern in such events may not necessarily explain the cause of death. However, it could well indicate whether one of the ingredients of the procedure which involves at least two components (cervical dilatation and uterine evacuation), can be absolved from blame.

Proponents of vacuum aspiration of molar tissue irrespective of uterine size claim that, apart from being a rapid technique, the use of negative pressure limits dissemination of the trophoblast and reduces loss of blood to a minimum [7]. Stone and Bagshawe [7], in their otherwise excellent study on the need for chemotherapy following various methods of evacuation of hydatidiform moles, appear to confirm the reduced risk of a subsequent need for chemotherapy after vacuum aspiration. The main limitation of their data, however, is the absence of information on uterine size, particularly since others [1, 8] have indicated that the risk of persistent trophoblastic disease is greatest in patients who are large for dates. The authors duly acknowledge this limitation, but analyse the results of a large group of gynaecologists, most of whom are said to take 12 or 14 weeks uterine size as their normal limit for vaginal termination of pregnancy. Hence, their apparent demonstration of a lower incidence of chemotherapy following vacuum aspiration is not likely to be representative for the type of second trimester molar pregnancy that is discussed here.

The argumentation that it is mainly the use of negative pressure that limits dissemination of trophoblast has a ring of logic, but does not quite differentiate fact from fancy. A study (unpublished) in our department has shown that vacuum aspiration of normal pregnancies in the early second trimester may result in a substantial release of foetal red cells into the maternal circulation. This may not necessarily relate to the question of dissemination of trophoblast in the maternal circulation during the evacuation of molar pregnancy. However, it shows that the use of negative pressure certainly does not prevent the occurrence of foeto-maternal transfusion. Furthermore, if there is such a marked effect of negative pressure in respect of trophoblast embolisation as one is often led to believe, one might expect two further findings. Firstly, vacuum aspiration should lead to a significantly lower incidence of subsequent chemotherapy than mere dilatation and curettage. The study of Stone and Bagshawe [7] showed that this was not the case. Secondly, since spontaneous abortion of a hydatidiform mole is more the result of positive than of negative intra-uterine pressure, one would expect that the need for chemotherapy would be significantly higher in this group. Again this was not so. Especially for spontaneous abortions at gestational ages of either less than 12 or less than 14 weeks, there was a subsequent need for chemotherapy in 5% of cases as compared to 4.5% in the entire vacuum aspiration group said to be mostly limited to uterine sizes of 12 – 14 weeks.

Therefore we can only conclude that there is no adequate evidence that a lower incidence of chemotherapy after vacuum aspiration is causally related to that particular method. On the contrary, there are ample indications that it relates more to the characteristics of the hydatidiform mole, such as uterine size, that induce the gynaecologist to select this particular mode of evacuation.

*Vacuum aspiration with myometrial stimulation*

Some authors [1] have advocated concomitant therapy with oxytocic drugs in association with vacuum aspiration, but others [7] claim that it may increase the risk of trophoblast embolisation. Much of the argumentation in favour of either of these approaches is poorly substantiated or inferred from general knowledge on uterine physiology and pharmacology. Some consider that prior myometrial stimulation is necessary to reduce the risk of uterine perforation and haemorrhage [9]. For others, uterine stimulation during or at the end of the evacuation should be adequate to achieve these aims. Stone and Bagshawe [7], however, specifically state that 'trophoblast embolisation is likely to be increased if ergometrine is given at the time of vacuum aspiration' but provide no data or references to substantiate that statement. Presumably, this opinion is a generalisation based on their observation of a lower need for subsequent chemotherapy after vacuum aspiration than after medical induction. If, and this is not certain, the above opinions on the necessity or desirability of uterine stimulation are true, such a statement may be potentially damaging, particularly when it is applied to other uterine stimulants as well. On the other hand, if that statement can be substantiated, it may throw a totally different light on the use of oxytocic drugs combined with vacuum aspiration.

However, that question is unlikely to be resolved within the next few years. It should be realised that, as mentioned above, the study of Stone and Bagshawe is based on the reports of a large number of gynaecologists who have used different approaches. From the study it is not clear whether the use of vacuum aspiration automatically implied that oxytocic drugs were not used at the time of uterine evacuation. This is unlikely to be the case, since 15% of the 611 patients underwent vacuum aspiration and 26.5% medical induction as the primary mode of evacuation, but apparently none a combination of these approaches. It is very unlikely that a large body of gynaecologists choosing medical induction as the primary treatment for as many as 26.5% of their patients, would have considered oxytocic drugs as sufficiently dangerous to systematically withhold these from the patients who underwent vacuum aspiration. Moreover, from the data it is not possible to exclude the possibility that the lower need for chemotherapy after vacuum aspiration may have occurred especially in those cases that received a myometrial stimulant at the time of uterine evacuation. That situation would be exactly the reverse of what is being claimed, and it emphasizes the need for carefully controlled studies in order to distinguish fact from fancy with regard to the use of myometrial stimulants in association with vacuum aspiration.

*Oxytocin*

It is well known that the uterus in midpregnancy is rather insensitive to oxytocin. In general, there is little response to oxytocin infusion before 20 weeks [10]. Beyond 20 weeks there is an increase in oxytocin sensitivity but then there is considerable individual variation in the uterine response to oxytocin. There has been much speculation about the reasons for the increasing sensitivity to oxytocin. This has been related to the level of spontaneous activity [11]. Owing to data on experimental animals showing an increase in oxytocin-induced contractility under the influence of progesterone withdrawal [12] and an increase in capacity and affinity of oxytocin binding sites under the influence of oestrogens [13], much attention has been given to hormonal changes. Little of this appears to be relevant to molar pregnancy, except for the possibility that it may be necessary to consider whether the hormonal characteristics of such pregnancies [14] could induce a greater sensitivity to oxytocin at an earlier stage in pregnancy. So far there are no indications that this is the case. Furthermore, from the available data on hormone concentrations in molar pregnancy, one might even expect the reverse to be true. Indeed, levels of plasma progesterone in patients with a molar pregnancy are usually found to be either similar [14] or elevated [15] in comparison with levels in normal pregnancy at corresponding gestational ages. Oestrogen excretion [16] and plasma levels [14], on the other hand, are generally lower than in women of similar gestational age but this is not always the case. Some authors [15] even found mean plasma levels of oestradiol-17$\beta$, the most potent compound, to be higher in molar pregnancy than in normal pregnancy of similar duration, whereas others [14] observed an opposite pattern. Nevertheless, it should be realised that the influence of hormone changes on uterine activity remains controversial even in normal pregnancy [17].

As the effectiveness of oxytocin is related to the level of spontaneous uterine contractility [10] and the ripeness of the cervix [18], very high doses are necessary in the earlier stages of pregnancy. Since Loudon [3] introduced the use of high doses of oxytocin to stimulate abortion of molar pregnancies in 1959, this approach has been used in a great many cases and with a certain degree of success. However, oxytocin can also cause maternal complications because of its anti-diuretic action which increases with the dose. At a dose of 45 mU/min its effect is said to equal that of vasopressin [10]. When given in large doses water intoxication can develop with generalised hypertonus, fits and unconsciousness, a potentially lethal complication. There is evidence that the risk of convulsions relates to the degree of hyponatraemia, the critical value for plasma sodium concentrations probably being 120 – 125 mmol/l [10]. These sodium concentrations can occur after as little as 4 l of dextrose in association with high doses of oxytocin [19].

In general, there appears to be a growing consensus of opinion now that oxytocin is not effective enough as a primary method for emptying the uterus in pregnancies complicated by hydatidiform mole [10]. This seems to be based on at least three grounds: the relative insensitivity of the midpregnant uterus to oxytocin, the maternal risks of excessive oxytocin dosage and the fact that, with the prostaglandins, better oxytocic drugs have become available to deal with early pregnancy in particular. On the other hand, as mentioned above, high doses of oxytocin for short periods of time are still used, in many centres, in association with vacuum aspiration to limit risks of perforation and haemorrhage. Others have used oxytocin in association with either systemic [20] or local [21] administration of prostaglandins in order to achieve a summation of the uterotonic effects [22]. In doing so, the dosage of the latter drug can be markedly reduced, which will result in a lower incidence and severity of gastro-intestinal side-effects [23].

*Prostaglandins*

In contrast to oxytocin, prostaglandins have the ability to induce uterine contractility at virtually all stages of pregnancy [22]. Furthermore they can be administered in almost every conceivable manner, although there are basically two options: local (intra-amniotic, extra-amniotic, etc.) or systemic (intravenous, oral, etc.) administration. Vaginal administration is occasionally considered as a local or a combined route of administration, but from the required doses and the obtained effects it is clear that it should be considered as a systemic administration, the effect of which depends on systemic absorption through the mucosae.

Since Karim [5] first reported on the use of $PGE_2$ for terminating molar pregnancy in 1970, both $PGE_2$ and $PGF_{2\alpha}$ have been used in different formulations and by various routes to terminate such pregnancies. It is now clearly established that both these prostaglandins are highly effective for stimulating abortion of a hydatidiform mole [9]. Almost independent of the route of administration or the duration of pregnancy, $PGE_2$ is about ten times more potent than $PGF_{2\alpha}$ [22, 23]. However the route of administration is a major issue to be considered in relation to molar pregnancy.

In general, with natural prostaglandins and in the second trimester of pregnancy, local administration is preferred (Craft, chapter 11), for two reasons in particular. Firstly, the natural prostaglandins have a short half-life in the circulation and over 90% of the drug administered may be inactivated by a single passage through the lungs [24]. Secondly, the high doses that are required in comparison to term pregnancy to stimulate the midtrimester uterus, result in a high incidence of side-effects. In practice this has resulted in a general preference for either intra-amniotic or extra-amniotic routes of administration in the second trimester of pregnancy (Craft, chapter 11). However, this does not nor can it apply to molar pregnancy. In such pregnancies amniotic fluid, amniotic membranes and consequently intra-amniotic and extra-amniotic spaces do not exist. Both the usual intra-amniotic and extra-amniotic approaches therefore result in a rather similar, unpredictable intra-uterine or intervesicular administration.

In the usual intra-amniotic administration amniotic fluid acts as a depot. The prostaglandins pass slowly across the foetal membranes and placenta to the uterus which is gradually stimulated. Compared to the extra-amniotic approach high doses are therefore required to compensate for dilution, transport through the membranes and active catabolism by the foetal membranes and placenta which have a high potential for prostaglandin inactivation from early in pregnancy [25]. In molar pregnancy all of this is disturbed. From amniographhy, employed at one time for radiological confirmation of hydatidiform mole, it is known that there is an instantaneous migration of the dye through the intervesicular septa, followed by prompt absorption into the systemic circulation. Hence, as pointed out by Karim [26], it is not surprising that neglecting these important considerations will result in severe systemic reactions. It may be reassuring that a so-called intra-amniotic administration of 20 mg $PGE_2$ in molar pregnancy [27] did not prove fatal, but it does not constitute optimal management. Clearly, there can be no room for the classical intra-amniotic administration (Craft, chapter 11) in molar pregnancy. In fact in other pregnancies too, every effort should be made to rule out hydatidiform mole when the intra-amniotic technique is resorted to for termination of pregnancy. Injection should be withheld if no free flow of amniotic fluid is obtained after puncture of the uterine cavity.

In respect of the so-called extra-amniotic techniques (see Craft, chapter 11) it is not possible to be so conclusive. We [21] and many others [9] have used this approach, the largest well-documented series being reported by Calder et al. [28]. These authors successfully terminated 9 molar pregnancies with $PGE_2$ in a mean time of 12.6 hours with minimal side-effects [28]. McNicol and Gray [29], however, described a severe systemic reaction to transcervical administration of 0.2 mg $PGE_2$, and in general, published experience with this procedure remains rather limited. With this procedure too, anatomical relations remain important. On the one hand, administration is not confined to the extrachorial space but is intra-uterine or intervesicular, whatever that may mean in terms of either dilution or myometrial and general absorption. On the other hand, in comparison to placental tissue, hydatidiform molar tissue has been noted to have a severely depressed capacity to catabolise prostaglandins [30]. This too may need to be considered, especially since the foetal membranes and the chorion in particular have an even greater potential for prostaglandin catabolism than the high activity present in placental tissue [31, 32]. Hence, it is certainly not justified to include such cases in large series of other terminations of pregnancy and thereupon to conclude on the safety of this approach in molar pregnancy.

On the basis of the available evidence, it is not possible to condemn intra-uterine administration of prostaglandins in molar pregnancy at present. On the other hand, much more data, including the risks of dissemination of trophoblast, are required before it can be recommended for routine use.

Systemic administration of $PGE_2$ or $PGF_{2\alpha}$ by intravenous infusion will virtually always succeed in terminating molar pregnancy. With only a few exceptions [33] most published reports deal with less than half a dozen and often with single case histories [9]. Infusion rates vary greatly from one study to another, although they remain usually at or below 5 $\mu$g/min for $PGE_2$ and 50 $\mu$g/min for $PGF_{2\alpha}$. Mean total doses have ranged up to 3 mg for $PGE_2$ and 37 mg for $PGF_{2\alpha}$. In these studies it was not always the aim to achieve complete expulsion of all molar tissue. Some [3] aimed to obtain a suitable cervical dilatation of 1–3 cm for subsequent vacuum aspiration of a well-contracted uterus. According to some [34] this should be preferred to continuing medical induction until spontaneous expulsion occurs and may reduce the incidence of uterine haemorrhage, a potentially major problem in spontaneous or drug-induced abortion of molar pregnancies. Southern et al. [35] reported on a series of 27 molar pregnancies terminated by vaginal suppositories containing 20 mg $PGE_2$. The treatment was successful in 23 patients (85%) with a mean dose of 78 mg and a mean induction–expulsion interval of 11.2 hours. These results are certainly not superior to the experience with intravenous $PGE_2$ [9]. Vomiting, diarrhoea and a temperature elevation of 2° F (1.2° C) or more occurred in respectively 63, 30 and 22% of cases [35]. In addition, 5 of these patients had a loss of blood of 1000 ml or more but 14 received a blood transfusion, though one of them before the prostaglandin therapy. One patient (3.7%) subsequently developed choriocarcinoma and was treated by hysterectomy and chemotherapy. Amy [34], discussing this report, suggested that aspiration of the uterine contents at a cervical dilatation of 3 cm or more could possibly have prevented much of the excessive loss of blood. This would seem to be a logical approach, particularly since the $PGE_2$ therapy was always followed by a diagnostic curettage [35]. However, there are no hard data to indicate whether that approach can reduce both the disadvantages of prostaglandin therapy and the aforementioned risks of vacuum aspiration. While the effectiveness of the natural prostaglandins for terminating molar pregnancy is now beyond doubt, the desirability and the actual benefit of their use in this condition will require further investigation.

*Prostaglandin analogues*

If anatomical considerations tend to favour systemic rather than intra-uterine administration of prostaglandins, prostaglandin analogues with a longer half-life and preferably a higher uterotonic specificity become a logical choice in molar pregnancy, more so than in other second trimester pregnancies (Amy, chapter 12).

So far, only a few reports have dealt with the use of prostaglandin analogues in molar pregnancy and not all have used systemic administration. One of the first reports actually dealt with transcervical intra-uterine administration of a $PGE_2$ analogue, 15(S)15-methyl-$PGE_2$ methyl ester, in 20 cases of molar pregnancy [36]. The results of a few studies that have used intravenous or intramuscular administration of various prostaglandin analogues are summarised in Table 1. The largest series of 23 cases was reported by Fawzy and Basiony [37], using 16-phenoxy-$\omega$-tetranor-$PGE_2$-methylsulphonylamide (sulprostone), but gestational ages, total doses and abortion intervals were not given separately for molar pregnancies as compared to other cases, and loss of blood was not reported. None of the remaining 34 patients in Table 1 had a loss of blood in excess of 700 ml. Only 2 (6.1%) lost 500 ml or more, as compared to an incidence of 48% after vaginal $PGE_2$ [35]. Termination of pregnancy was, to some extent, successful in all cases, but in one study [37] this related to a cervical dilatation of 2 cm or more and in another [40] it includes two patients who had vacuum aspiration at a cervical dilatation of 10 mm or more. Gastro-intestinal side-effects remain a major issue to contend with, as in other second trimester terminations (Amy, chapter 12).

*Uterine stimulants in general*

The use of uterine stimulants in general as a primary method for the evacuation of hydatidiform moles has been brought into disrepute by Stone and Bagshawe [7], who demonstrated a higher need for chemotherapy after medical induction with oxytocin and/or prostaglandins than after spontaneous abortion, dilatation and curettage or vacuum aspiration. In the discussion of vauum aspiration it was already emphasised that there may be considerable bias in that study, but this does not allow us to ignore its implications entirely. On the other hand, from the above it can be estimated how heterogeneous a group of medical inductions may be, particularly when this is based not on a standard strategy but on analysis of the reports of a large number of gynaecologists. Considering the availability of oxytocic drugs in the United Kingdom, it is likely that this group consisted of oxytocin administration and of the administration of natural prostaglandins either as an intravenous infusion or in various forms of intra-uterine administration. It is not known whether insertion of, or injections through, an intra-uterine catheter may influence dissemination of trophoblast. However, it should be clear that one cannot conveniently combine all of these different approaches into one group and thereby hope to arrive at a valid evaluation of risk against benefit.

From the study of Stone and Bagshawe [7] it is also not clear whether medical induction was routinely followed by vacuum aspiration and/or curettage in order to ensure that the uterine cavity had been emptied completely.

*Table 1* Termination of molar pregnancy by systemic administration of prostaglandin analogues

| No of patients | Gestation in weeks | Uterine size in weeks | Prostaglandin | Dose | Route | Mean abortion interval (h min) | References |
|---|---|---|---|---|---|---|---|
| 14 | 11 – 16 | 18 – 28 | 2a, 2b-dihomo-15 (S)-methyl-$PGF_{2\alpha}$ methyl ester | 0 5 mg every 8h | Intra-muscular | 12 34 | Karim and Ratnam [38] |
| 9 | 11 – 16 | 14 – 22 | 16-phenoxy-ω-17, 18,19,20-tetranor-$PGE_2$ methyl sulphonyl-amide | 0 5 mg every 6h | Intra-muscular | 11 05 | Karim et al [39] |
| 23 | ? | ? | 16-phenoxy-ω-17, 18,19,20-tetranor-$PGE_2$ methyl sulphonyl-amide | 83 3 μg/h | Intravenous infusion | ? | Fawzy and Basiony [37] |
| 11 | 9 – 24 | 15 – 24 | 15(S)-methyl-$PGF_{2\alpha}$ | 0 25 mg every 2h | Intra-muscular | 15 40 | Keirse [40] |

That is another factor that may greatly influence the need for subsequent chemotherapy. Considering the gross appearance of hydatidiform moles, it is generally not possible to ensure that evacuation has been complete without exploration of the uterine cavity. Therefore, most authors consider routine vacuum and/or conventional curettage as essential following medically induced evacuation, whether judged to be complete or not [33, 34, 40].

Condemning uterine stimulants on the basis of the evidence presented [7] would certainly not be justified. It could be potentially dangerous or damaging, if the immediate risks [9] of vacuum aspiration of a large uterus are not over-stated or if this implies a return to hysterotomy and/or hysterectomy for the large uterine sizes. Therefore, a firm disavowal of the recent study of Stone and Bagshawe would be required if that study did not, in addition to many other positive features, raise the crucial question of what should be achieved by terminating molar pregnancy. Most studies on the use of uterine stimulants, including our own [21, 40] have devoted attention mainly, if not exclusively, to immediate efficacy, with little consideration of the subsequent follow-up. Some reports [35, 38] have referred to the subsequent development of choriocarcinoma in one or more patients, but there has been no consistent effort to include the long-term prognosis as an integral part in the evaluation of uterine stimulants for terminating second trimester molar pregnancy.

So far many reports on the use of uterine stimulants, whether it be oxytocin [3, 20], prostaglandins [20, 21, 34] or prostaglandin analogues [37], have been included in series of terminations of pregnancy conducted for reasons of foetal death, foetal abnormality or unwanted pregnancy. Such combined data may provide information on the uterotonic activity of the compound under study, but they are generally useless for examining its value in molar pregnancy. Indeed, such studies usually judge termination of a molar pregnancy by the same criteria applied to and made for other pregnancies, thereby ignoring all of the specific features of molar pregnancy. The first consequence of it usually consists of a total lack of information on subsequent follow-up and need for chemotherapy. Success is often judged in terms of complete and incomplete expulsion, a distinction that is rather irrelevant in molar pregnancy, since most authors agree that instrumental emptying of the uterine cavity is mandatory, whatever degree of completeness may be achieved. Furthermore, a compound that, for instance, effects a cervical dilatation of 2–3 cm within 2 hours in about 90% of cases may be a poor abortifacient and still be superior for terminating molar pregnancy to another one that has no such effect but achieves expulsion in 85% of cases within 24 hours. Possibly the aim should not be to achieve expulsion of all or most molar tissue, but to obtain a cervical dilatation and/or uterine contractility that allows mechanical evacuation with a minimum of risks [40].

CONCLUSIONS

At present it is not possible to assess adequately the merits and hazards of various methods for terminating second trimester molar pregnancy. As mentioned above several criticisms can and have been voiced against all of our currently favoured methods. These criticisms have two main characteristics in common. Firstly, they are serious in that they include sudden maternal deaths due to vacuum aspiration, an increased risk of dissemination of trophoblast by using oxytocic drugs in association with this procedure and a higher need for chemotherapy after medical induction. Secondly, they are all poorly documented and may not necessarily stand up to closer scrutiny. Under these circumstances it can hardly be surprising that recommending either one of these procedures mainly relates to one's personal fancies, irrespective of whether or not they can be supported by the most holy of clinical facts, i.e. "in my experience such dreadful complications do not occur". This is not too serious, for most clinicians will be aware of the scientific merit (or lack thereof) of such statements of fact. The potential hazards are far greater when such fancies result in an unwarranted prejudice against a particular method. Whereas the former approach may stimulate people to gather adequate data in support of that fancy, the latter actively discourages such endeavours.

In view of the conflicting evidence, the only way to assess adequately which of the above approaches provides the best benefit to risk ratio appears to be a carefully designed prospective study. Such a study will need to consider both immediate and long-term risks and benefits in cases that are adequately matched for gestational age and uterine size and randomly allocated to any one of two or three groups. Considering our experience [40] and the incidence of molar pregnancy in Western societies, it is not likely that the results of such a trial will be forthcoming in the near future. At present this should form no bar to the collection of adequate and thoroughly valid facts in support of whatever fancy. It may well prove to be a more fruitful approach than to depend on some statements of fact, merely to achieve a collection of largely unsubstantiated fancies.

REFERENCES

1. Curry SL, Hammond CB, Tyrey L, Creasman WT and Parker RT: Hydatidiform mole. Diagnosis, management and long-term follow-up of 347 patients. *Obstet Gynecol* 45: 1–8, 1975.
2. Surwit EA and Hammond CB: Gestational trophoblastic neoplasia. In: *Year Book of Obstetrics and Gynecology 1980*, Pitkin RM and Zlatnik FJ (eds), pp. 275–293. Year Book Medical Publishers, Chicago-London, 1980.
3. Loudon JDO: The use of high concentration oxytocin intravenous drips in the management of missed abortion. *J Obstet Gynaecol Br Empire* 66: 277–281, 1959.

4 Brandes JM, Grunstein S and Peretz A Suction evacuation of the uterine cavity in hydatidiform mole *Obstet Gynecol* 28 689–691, 1966

5 Karim SMM The use of prostaglandin $E_2$ in the management of missed abortion, missed labour and hydatidiform mole *Br Med J* 3 196–197, 1970

6 Ratnam SS and Honofia Medan J cited by Karim et al (9)

7 Stone M and Bagshawe KD An analysis of the influences of maternal age, gestational age, contraceptive method, and the mode of primary treatment of patients with hydatidiform moles on the incidence of subsequent chemotherapy *Br J Obstet Gynaecol* 86 782–792, 1979

8 Morrow CP, Kletzky OA, Disaia PJ, Townsend DE, Mishell DR and Nakamura RM Clinical and laboratory correlates of molar pregnancy and trophoblastic disease *Am J Obstet Gynecol* 128 424–430, 1977

9 Karim SMM, Ng SC and Ratnam SS Termination of abnormal intrauterine pregnancy with prostaglandins *Practical Applications of Prostaglandins and their Synthesis Inhibitors*, Karim SMM (ed), pp 319–374 MTP, Lancaster, 1979

10 Turnbull AC Influencing uterine contractility with oxytocin *Human Parturition New Concepts and Developments*, Keirse MJNC, Anderson ABM and Bennebroek Gravenhorst J (eds), pp 143–153 Leiden University Press, The Hague, 1979

11 Anderson ABM and Turnbull AC Spontaneous contractility and oxytocin sensitivity of the human uterus in mid-pregnancy *J Obstet Gynaecol Br Commonw* 75 271–277, 1968

12 Fuchs AR Parturition in rats and rabbits *Mem Soc Endocrinol* 20 163–186, 1973

13 Soloff MS Uterine receptor for oxytocin effects of estrogen *Biochem Biophys Res Commun* 65 205–212, 1975

14 Mochizuki M, Morikawa H, Kawaguchi K and Tojo S Growth hormone, prolactine and chorionic somatomammotropin in normal and molar pregnancy *J Clin Endocrinol Metab* 43 614–621, 1976

15 Chew PCT and Ratnam SS Steroid production in hydatidiform mole *Singapore J Obstet Gynaecol* 10 23–32, 1979

16 Frandsen VA and Stakeman G The excretion of hormones in cases of hydatidiform mole and chorionepithelioma *Acta Endocrinol Suppl* 90 81–88, 1964

17 Flint APF Role of progesterone and oestrogens in the control of the onset of labour in man a continuing controversy *Human Parturition New Concepts and Developments*, Keirse MJNC, Anderson ABM and Bennebroek Gravenhorst J (eds), pp 85–100 Leiden University Press, The Hague, 1979

18 Calder AA The management of the unripe cervis *Human Parturition New Concepts and Developments*, Keirse MJNC, Anderson ABM and Bennebroek Gravenhorst J (eds), pp 201–217 Leiden University Press, The Hague, 1979

19 Morgan DB, Kirwan NA, Hancock KW, Robinson D and Ahman S Water intoxication and oxytocin infusion *Br J Obstet Gynaecol* 84 6–12, 1977

20 Naismith WCMK and Barr W Simultaneous intravenous infusion of prostaglandin $E_2$ ($PGE_2$) and oxytocin in the management of intrauterine death of the fetus, missed abortion and hydatidiform mole *J Obstet Gynaecol Br Commonw* 81 146–149, 1974

21 Luengo J, Keirse MJNC and Bennebroek Gravenhorst J Extra-amniotic prostaglandin $F_{2\alpha}$ for intra uterine death and fetal abnormality *Eur J Obstet Gynecol Reprod Biol* 7 325–329, 1977

22 Embrey MP *Prostaglandins in reproduction* Churchill, London, 1975

23 Thiery M Induction of labor with prostaglandins *Human Parturition New Concepts and Developments*, Keirse MJNC, Anderson ABM and Bennebroek Gravenhorst J (eds), pp 155–164 Leiden University Press, The Hague, 1979

24 Ferreira SH and Vane JR Prostaglandins their disappearance from and release into the circulation *Nature* 216 868–873, 1967

25 Keirse MJNC, Williamson JG and Turnbull AC Metabolism of prostaglandin $F_{2\alpha}$ within the human uterus in early pregnancy *Br J Obstet Gynaecol* 82 142–145, 1975

26 Karim SMM Adverse reactions to intra-amniotic prostaglandin *Br Med J* 3 347, 1974

27 Smith AM Adverse reactions to intra-amniotic prostaglandins *Br Med J* 2 382–383, 1974

28  Calder AA, MacKenzie IZ and Embrey MP  Intrauterine (extraamniotic) prostaglandins in the management of unsuccessful pregnancy  *J  Reprod Med* 16  271–275, 1976

29  McNicol E and Gray H  Adverse reaction to extra-amniotic prostaglandin $E_2$  *Br J Obstet Gynaecol* 84  229–230, 1977

30  Alam NA, Clary P and Russell PT  Depressed placental prostaglandin $E_1$ metabolism in toxemia of pregnancy  *Prostaglandins* 4  363–370, 1973

31  Keirse MJNC and Turnbull AC  Metabolism of prostaglandins within the pregnant uterus  *Br J Obstet Gynaecol* 82  887–893, 1975

32  Keirse MJNC, Hanssens MCAJA, Hicks BR and Turnbull AC  Prostaglandin metabolism in placenta and chorion before and after the onset of labor  *Eur J Obstet Gynecol Reprod Biol* 6  1–5, 1976

33  Klausch B, Kruse HJ, Goretzlehner G and Buttner HH  Weheninduktion mit Prostaglandin $F_{2\alpha}$ zur Behandlung der Blasenmole  *Zentralbl Gynakol* 98  1352–1355, 1976

34  Amy JJ  Interruption de grossesse provoquee par les prostaglandines  In  *Les Prostaglandines et la Reproduction Humaine*, Amy JJ (ed), pp 141–173  Flammarion, Paris, 1979

35  Southern EM, Gutknecht GD and Mohberg NR  Evacuation of the uterus in benign gestational trophoblastic disease with prostaglandins  *Obstetric and Gynecological Uses of Prostaglandins*, Karim SMM (ed), pp 247–251  Asian Fed Obstet Gynecol, Singapore, 1976

36  Karim SMM, Ratnam SS and Choo HT  Intrauterine administration of prostaglandin 15(S)-15-methyl-$E_2$-methyl ester in the management of patients with a hydatidiform mole  *J Obstet Gynaecol Br Commonw* 81  650–651, 1974

37  Fawzy A and Basiony BA  The use of sulprostone in the management of death in utero and molar pregnancy  *Singapore J Obstet Gynaecol* 10  39–42, 1979

38  Karim SMM and Ratnam SS  Termination of abnormal intrauterine pregnancies with intramuscular administration of dihomo-15-methyl prostaglandin $F_{2\alpha}$  *Br J Obstet Gynaecol* 83  885–889, 1976

39  Karim SMM, Lim AL, Prasad RNV, Yeo KC, Ng, SC, Salmon YM, Choo HT and Ratnam SS  Termination of abnormal intrauterine pregnancy with intramuscular administration of sulprostone  *Singapore J Obstet Gynaecol* 10  33–37, 1979

40  Keirse MJNC  Termination of molar pregnancy by intramuscular administration of 15(S)-15-methyl-prostaglandin $F_{2\alpha}$  *Prostaglandins Med* 4  333–339, 1980

# 11. NATURAL PROSTAGLANDINS ALONE OR IN COMBINATION FOR TERMINATION OF PREGNANCY

### IAN CRAFT

The first report of the successful use of natural prostaglandins for termination of pregnancy [1] occurred at a time established pharmacological methods were under criticism because of concern about their unpredictable response, the long time to abortion and the degree of morbidity and mortality resulting from the use of various agents. There was particular concern about reports of severe sepsis following the use of hypertonic glucose and of occasional fatalities from cerebral infarction resulting from misadministration of hypertonic saline. The role of prostaglandins for the management of midtrimester abortion was evaluated in clinical trials utilizing different routes of administration with the aim of achieving complete abortion by a single procedure without the need for other procedures or stimulants. An ever-decreasing time to abortion came to be seen as the most critical index of a particular technique or method of administration, and as a consequence some methods appeared to have limitations which led, on the one hand, to their restricted usage and, on the other hand, to modification of techniques and to combination therapy.

Whilst women in the midtrimester exhibit varied 'inducibility' features, akin to those assessed in late pregnancy by the Bishop's score, it is understandable that some techniques may cause adverse consequences from excessive myometrial activity when a fixed dose is used which cannot be altered once it has been injected, or because oxytocin is given for apparent limited response.

Although the objective of finding a method which is invariably effective within a reasonable time, preferably non-invasive, and without side-effects remains elusive, it has been possible with time to develop natural prostaglandin techniques towards this end.

### NATURAL PROSTAGLANDINS

The success of using prostaglandins is influenced by the nature of the prostaglandin given ($PGE_2$ or $PGF_{2\alpha}$), the dosage (single or repeated), the preparation (solution, pessary, gel, etc.), the route of administration, the gestational length, and whether augmentation is used (laminaria, oxytocin, etc.).

Oral therapy is ineffective at this gestation and intramuscular usage is irritant. Pessary administration is appealing because it is non-invasive and would allow in some situations supervision by non-medical personnel. Variable side-effects and success rates have been reported in different studies which are probably related in part to the formulation used. Elias [2] described only limited success with a high incidence of fever and gastro-intestinal problems, whilst others [3, 4] using $PGE_2$ 20 mg pessaries every 2–4 h reported excellent success in a mean time of approximately 12 h (range 5.5–35.5). In 8 of the 40 patients treated the membranes ruptured spontaneously and the prostaglandin pessaries were stopped; uterine activity being augmented with intravenous oxytocin [4]. Vomiting and/or diarrhoea occurred in 30 patients (75%) with repeated episodes occurring in 24 women. A temperature rise of 100° F was noted in 55%.

Whilst Karim and Filshie [1] first described the successful use of intravenous prostaglandins with 14 of 15 pregnancies being terminated following administration of $PGF_{2\alpha}$ 50 $\mu$g/min, approximately 50% of the patients vomited and/or had diarrhoea. With $PGE_2$ 5$\mu$g/min [5] abortion resulted in 50 out of 52 patients and gastro-intestinal symptoms occurred in a smaller number, viz. 14. Embrey [6] succeeded in terminating 28 out of 30 patients with an infusion of $PGE_2$ 2–5 $\mu$g/min. Only 5 patients vomited and none had diarrhoea. Other studies have indicated that the induction – abortion interval may be prolonged, and that side-effects are troublesome with higher doses. The latter was noted particularly by Hillier and Embrey [7] when doses of up to $PGE_2$ 20 $\mu$g/min and $PGF_{2\alpha}$ 200 $\mu$g/min were administered. It was also found that there was no increase in success rate with an increase of the infusion dose; indeed, the reverse was found. Subsequently Coltart and Coe [8] described the beneficial effects of administering concomittant oxytocin given at 128 mU/min following a 2-h priming period with prostaglandin $E_2$ given up to a maximum dose of 10 $\mu$g/min. All 19 patients treated in this fashion aborted in a mean time of 16 h and only one patient took longer than 24 h. Vomiting occurred in 13 cases (68%) and there was a tendency for superficial phlebitis to be observed along the infusion vein.

Intra-amniotic prostaglandin usage requires careful amniocentesis following placental localization by ultrasound and is only suitable for pregnancies beyond 15 weeks gestation. It is preferable if injections are made via an indwelling catheter rather than through a needle, thereby minimizing possible misadministration and consequent systemic effects of injecting the agent outside the gestation sac (e.g. bronchoconstriction). Karim and Sharma [9] reported success in each patient treated with one injection of either $PGE_2$ 2.5–5.0 mg or $PGF_{2\alpha}$ 25 mg in a study of 10 patients. Yet, a larger evaluation indicated that when increasing single doses of prostaglandin are given up to a maximum of $PGE_2$ 20 mg or $PGF_{2\alpha}$ 100 mg, abortion is not invariably successful within 24 h of a single injection, although there is a dose response relationship with mean times to abortion of 13 and $17\frac{1}{2}$ h respectively [10]. With $PGE_2$ 20 mg diarrhoea occurred in 23% of the cases and vomiting in 46%. Other investigators assessed the efficacy of administering $PGF_{2\alpha}$ 25 mg and found a need to repeat the injections on one or more occasions. This dose repeated at 24 h produced a success rate of 97% in a mean time of 28 h [11]. Success rates varying from 70 to 100% have been reported using a single injection of 40–50 mg $PGF_{2\alpha}$ with a mean time to abortion varying between 16 and 25 h. Results of these investigations led the Upjohn Company to formulate proposals for the intra-amniotic route whereby $PGE_2$ was administered as a stat dose of 10 mg and $PGF_{2\alpha}$ 40 mg to be repeated at 24 h if abortion had not occurred or was not progressing satisfactorily towards completion by that time. Besides gastro-intestinal stimulation, other sequelae described include bronchoconstriction if the agent gained rapid access to the systemic circulation, occasionally seen when a needle rather than a catheter was used, and of cervical injuries occurring in up to 3% of patients, especially in nulliparae where excessive doses may have been used and in those receiving oxytocin. Whilst coagulopathy has not been found to be a problem with this method, foetal viability in pregnancies of advanced gestation has caused concern.

The principles of correct management of the patient include adequate explanation of the procedure, preliminary ultrasound for placental localization and confirmation of gestation, suitable analgesia for the amniocentesis and for subsequent uterine contractility (I have previously reported on the beneficial effects of epidural analgesia, especially in the young) and regular vaginal assessments to monitor progress. Anti-D is necessary for all Rhesus negative patients and routine uterine examination allows assessment of the cervical status and ensures there is no retained placental tissue.

Extra-amniotic therapy has an advantage in practice over intra-amniotic application in that it is applicable from 12 weeks onwards and not restricted to after 15 weeks. Total dose required is less than with intravenous use and the side-effects are relatively few with occasional diarrhoea, vomiting and fever. Prostaglandins may be administered in solution or gel form. With the former instillation may be done intermittently via an indwelling catheter every few hours or by continuous pump administration. The success rate using $PGF_{2\alpha}$ 750 $\mu$g every 2-h was approximately 70% in a mean time of 24 h with comparable rates using $PGE_2$ 200 $\mu$g in 19 h [11, 12]. Miller et al. [13] reported a success rate of 90% with a continuous $PGE_2$ infusion in a mean time of 15.75 h (range 6–30 h) with a low incidence of side-effects. Midwinter et al. [14] assessed the effectiveness of various infusion rates and dosages and reported that $PGE_2$ 66–133 $\mu$g/hr resulted in abortion within 36 h of 61 out of 68 patients. With a lower dose of 46 $\mu$g/hr the mean injection-abortion interval increased and only 13 out of 20 patients so treated aborted within this time.

Sice-effects were limited with higher dosages. There is generally considered to be a lower incidence of cervical injury with extra-amniotic application than with intra-amniotic use but Krishna et al. [15] have reported a 2.4% incidence with $PGF_{2\alpha}$ 750 μg given every 2 h. Some of the disparity between the incidence of cervical lacerations being reported in different studies may depend upon whether evacuation and cervical inspection is performed as a routine on all patients treated.

High dose prostaglandins suspended in an appropriate viscous gel, e.g. Tylose, allow a gradual release with time with a relatively low incidence of systemic side-effects. Lippert and Modly [16] were the first to report excellent success with intermittent injections of $PGE_2$ 1.25 mg or $PGF_{2\alpha}$ 3.75 mg given every 2–3 h via an indwelling catheter. Abortion occurred in each of 20 patients treated, with a mean injection–abortion interval of 11.5 h in those receiving $PGE_2$ and 17.6 h in those receiving $PGF_{2\alpha}$. Only 5 patients experienced any vomiting. Subsequently, MacKenzie and Embrey [17] advocated using a single dose of $PGE_2$ 1.5–3.0 mg with removal of the insertion catheter following instillation of the prostaglandins and reported a success rate of 70% within 24 h. They evaluated the efficacy of using different doses of $PGE_2$, viz. 1.0 mg, 1.5 mg, 2.0 mg or 3.0 mg and found no increase in success rate above 75% when doses of 1.5 mg or more were injected. There was, however, a dose-dependent association with the incidence of gastro-intestinal side-effects, which occurred in 70% of patients with the highest dose used. The mean injection–abortion interval was approximately 16 h with the most effective dose. Craft et al. [18] have reported limitations using a single injection and preferred to use $PGE_2$ 3.5 mg given every 6 h with the instillation catheter being withdrawn on each occasion. So far cervical injuries have not been observed in over 100 patients treated. Half the patients had one episode of vomiting but this was not troublesome and diarrhoea did not occur at this dose level, although it was observed in patients in whom $PGE_2$ 4.0 mg was assessed. Some adverse reaction may occur with this method of administration following systemic $PGE_2$ absorption if the catheter is inserted too far into the uterus and/or the instillation is made too rapidly. Side-effects that may be experienced include uterine cramps and sensations of respiratory difficulty, coldness and shivering, etc.

PROSTAGLANDIN COMBINATION METHODS

Various agents augment prostaglandin activity and result in less prostaglandin being required, an increased success rate with time, a shorter time to abortion, and in some a lower incidence of side-effects. However, some problems have been reported to occur including sepsis with laminaria tents, water intoxication with high dose oxytocin therapy, coagulopathy, tissue necrosis and occasional fatalities with hypertonic solutions and cervical lacerations following excessive uterine stimulation. An example of one intra-amniotic and one extra-amniotic method will be described.

## Extra-amniotic

The instillation of 150 ml of 0.1% Rivanol results in a mean time to abortion at 24 h, 48 h and 72 h of 29%, 77% and 88% of patients respectively. Martin et al. [19] reported an increased success rate in a shorter mean time when $PGF_{2\alpha}$ 750 $\mu g$ was infused extra-amniotically in the first hour after instillation of the Rivanol solution. More patients complained of pain and vomited with the combined method. Olund and Larsson [20] compared the efficacy of administering 0.1% Rivanol alone, $PGF_{2\alpha}$ alone (250 $\mu g$ stat followed by 750 $\mu g$ every 2 h) and Rivanol combined with $PGF_{2\alpha}$ in the above dosage and manner. The mean induction–abortion time in this study was similar in all groups. A number of patients given $PGF_{2\alpha}$ alone or in combination aborted earlier than patients given Rivanol alone. The balloon of the Foley catheter used was distended with 30 ml of solution as opposed to 10 ml in the Himmelman study [21]. Gastro-intestinal side-effects were common in all groups, but not significantly worse with those receiving prostaglandins.

## Intra-amniotic

Hypertonic urea was introduced as a potentially safer agent than hypertonic saline since it is used in certain medical emergencies, but it is relatively ineffective when injected alone as a solution containing 80 g with a mean injection–abortion interval of 59 h [22]. Intravenous high dose oxytocin augmentation may reduce this interval to approximately 20 h [23] but there may be rare sequelae in doing so, e.g. water intoxication especially if excessive amounts of electrolyte-free solutions are administered. In 1973 Craft [24] and Bowen-Simpkins [25] first reported the effects of injecting 80 g of urea solution combined with $PGE_2$ 5–10 mg. The abortion time was dramatically reduced to approximately 10 h following a single instillation only. All intra-amniotic procedures require careful amniocentesis and many advise removing a certain volume of liquor prior to injection of the urea solution. Whereas it had been previously demonstrated that intra-amniotic prostaglandins given in high doses result in a significant decrease in plasma sex steroid concentrations, even more marked changes were noted with urea and prostaglandin combinations and these were found to be significant as early as one hour after the injection procedure [26]. Using prostaglandin $E_2$ it was found possible to reduce the amount injected from 10 mg down to 5 mg and eventually to 2.5 mg without adversely affecting the success of a single shot procedure or the mean time to abortion. In addition $PGF_{2\alpha}$ given in a dose of 10 mg was found to be equally efficacious [27]. The presence of a dead foetus was recognized to be an advantage but other adverse effects gradually became apparent, including an increased incidence of vomiting and diarrhoea especially with the higher prostaglandin doses compared to when the same dose of prostaglandin was used alone, and in addition a 4.5% incidence of cervical laceration [28]. There have also been occasional reports of coagulopathy. It has recently been reported that the already short time to abortion can be even further reduced by the preliminary use of laminaria tents and/or intravenous oxytocin therapy [29].

CONCLUSIONS

During the past decade various modifications of prostaglandin administration have been evaluated by different groups. The author initially assessed the dose–response relationships of administering $PGE_2$ or $PGF_{2\alpha}$ in a single dose but appreciated that there are limitations to this application since some patients will require additional prostaglandin dosage or other stimulants to complete the abortion process. I also became increasingly concerned about the risk of cervical damage and its possible effect on subsequent desired pregnancies. Early assessment of the urea and prostaglandin technique appeared particularly favourable showing a reduction in the time to abortion as compared with intra-amniotic prostaglandins administered alone while ensuring lack of foetal viability. However, a cervical laceration rate of 4.5% is unacceptable, and because of this it was decided to pursue alternative techniques for routine use. It is now our practice to use extra-amniotic $PGE_2$ 3.5 mg in Tylose gel every 6 h since the efficacy appears to be better in overall terms than the prostaglandin and urea combination and our assessment of the results of using some of the new analogues. However, we have reluctantly reverted to using the urea and prostaglandin combination recently for pregnancies in excess of 20 weeks gestation to ensure lack of foetal viability and avoid any undue public or professional criticism.

I am aware of the debate as to the place of dilatation and evacuation as opposed to inductive methods and am particularly mindful of the psychological and traumatic effects of the latter technique. There is a need to prospectively assess both morbidity and mortality rates of the different approaches at comparable gestations including especially their effect on subsequent obstetric performance and the role of operator error in the different methods available for use.

REFERENCES

1  Karım SMM and Fılshıe GM  *Lancet* 1  157, 1970
2  Elıas JA  *Adv Bıoscı* 9  581, 1973
3  Lauerson NH, Secher MJ and Wılson KH  *Am J Obstet Gynecol* 122  947, 1975
4  Bolognese RJ and Corson SL  *Am J Obstet Gynecol* 120  281, 1974
5  Karım SMM and Fılshıe GM  *Br Med J* 3  198, 1970
6  Embrey MP  *J Reprod Med* 6  15, 1971
7  Hıllıer K and Embrey MP  *J Obstet Gynaecol Br Commonw* 79  14, 1972
8  Coltart TM and Coe MJ  *Lancet* 1  173, 1975
9  Karım SMM and Sharma D  *Lancet* 2  147, 1971
10  Craft I  *J Obstet Gynaecol Br Commonw* 80  46, 1973
11  BygdemanM, Begum F, Toppozada AM and Wıqvıst N  *Adv Bıoscı* 9  525, 1973
12  Embrey MP, Hıllıer K and Mahendran P  *Adv Bıoscı* 9  507, 1973
13  Mıller AWF, Calder AA and Macnaughton MC  *Lancet* 2  5, 1972
14  Mıdwınter A, Shepherd A and Bowen M  *J Obstet Gynaecol Br Commonw* 80  371, 1973
15  Krıshna U, Gangulı AC, Mandlekar AV and Purandare VN  *Prostaglandıns* 15  685, 1978
16  Lıppert TH and Modly T  *J Obstet Gynaecol Br Commonw* 80  1025, 1973
17  MacKenzıe IZ and Embrey MP  *Bı J Obstet Gynaecol* 83  505, 1976
18  Craft I, Evans D, Rıchfield L and Yovıch J  *Gynaecol Obstet Invest* 9  256, 1978
19  Martın JM, Bygdeman M, Leader A and Wıqvıst N  *Contraception* 11  523, 1975
20  Olund A and Larsson B  *Acta Obstet Gynecol Scand* 77  333, 1978
21  Hımmelmann A, Myhrıman P and Svanberg SG  *Contraception* 12  645, 1975
22  Greenhalf JO and Dıggory PLC  *Br Med J* 1  28, 1971
23  Craft I and Musa B  *Lancet* 2  1058, 1971
24  Craft I  *Lancet* 1  779, 1973
25  Bowen-Sımpkıns P  *J Obstet Gynaecol Br Commonw* 80  824, 1973
26  Craft IL, Fergusson ILC, Smıth B and Youssefnejadıan E  *J Obstet Gynaecol Br Commonw* 80  1095, 1973
27  Craft I, Walker E and Youssefnejadıan E  *Prostaglandıns,* 5  397, 1974
28  Craft I  *Lancet* 1  1115, 1975
29  Wılson WB  *Obstet Gynecol* 51  699, 1978

## 12. TERMINATION OF SECOND TRIMESTER PREGNANCY WITH PROSTAGLANDIN ANALOGUES

JEAN-JACQUES AMY

Although the naturally occurring prostaglandins provide a more effective and probably a safer means of terminating second trimester pregnancy than methods previously known, they still have some definite shortcomings. When given systemically, they frequently cause unacceptable side-effects. To avoid intolerance, natural prostaglandins are best instilled directly into the uterus, making use of either the extra- or the intra-amniotic route. Both techniques require expertise on the part of the attending obstetrician. Moreover, the chemicals are rapidly metabolized in vivo (except for the amniotic cavity) and it is necessary to administer repeat doses at short intervals or, on the contrary, a very large single dose.

For many years now, an intensive search has been underway in pharmaceutical laboratories, aiming at the synthesis of structurally modified analogues, which would display enhanced uterotonic specificity and greater resistance to metabolic inactivation. Early examples of such analogues, designed to resist $C_{15}$-dehydrogenation, are the 15-methyl and 16,16-dimethyl derivatives of $PGE_2$ and $PGF_{2\alpha}$. Both types of compounds have been widely studied as abortifacients. Both have their limitations. As was the case for the natural prostaglandins, the high frequency of side-effects caused by the 15-methyl analogues precludes to a point their systemic administration. The 16,16-dimethyl prostaglandins exhibit greater selectivity for the uterus. They therefore, lend themselves better to vaginal administration, which is technically easy and is more acceptable to the patient. However, 16,16-dimethyl prostaglandins are unstable in suppository form and this is a major obstacle to their large scale production.

Of the recently developed analogues, 16-phenoxy-$\omega$-17,18,19,20-tetranor-$PGE_2$-methylsulphonamide seems to be the most promising, yet it could be superseded within the next few years by compounds more selective still, suitable for oral administration.

$\omega$-HOMO-PGE$_1$

Gillespie, Beazley and Van Dorp[1] were the first, in 1971, to report on the use of an "unnatural" prostaglandin for induction of abortion. These authors succeeded in terminating two out of three midtrimester pregnancies by intravenously infusing 5–6.7 $\mu$g/min of $\omega$-homo-$PGE_1$. In the third case, oxytocin was required for completion of abortion. Side-effects were not reported. No further assessment of this compound was made.

## 20-ETHYL-$PGF_{2\alpha}$

Sharp and Burslem [2] were able to induce abortion in 5 out of 6 women at 9–17 weeks gestation by intravenously infusing 5–125 $\mu$g/min racemic 20-ethyl $PGF_{2\alpha}$. Every patient developed venous erythema at the site of infusion and also had many episodes of emesis and diarrhoea.

## $PGE_2$ METHYL ESTER

The abortifacient efficacy of $PGE_2$ methyl ester (Fig. 1) was evaluated by Karim and Amy [3] in 25 women at 12–24 weeks gestation. The drug was administered either by the intra-amniotic route (single dose of 2.5 mg) or the extra-amniotic route (250 $\mu$g; no second dose given because of intolerance). Given in sufficient dosage, $PGE_2$ methyl ester caused gastro-intestinal, central nervous and cardiovascular side-effects considerably more severe than those seen with $PGE_2$. One patient given 2.5 mg $PGE_2$ methyl ester vaginally developed an acute febrile encephalopathy requiring immediate treatment. Diarrhoea was more frequent than vomiting. Due to systemic absorption, side-effects were most severe after vaginal administration. But, whatever the route of delivery used, side-effects appeared within a few minutes, indicating prompt passage of the compound into the circulation. The drug unquestionably did not compare favourably with the natural prostaglandins or other analogues, and it was not assessed further.

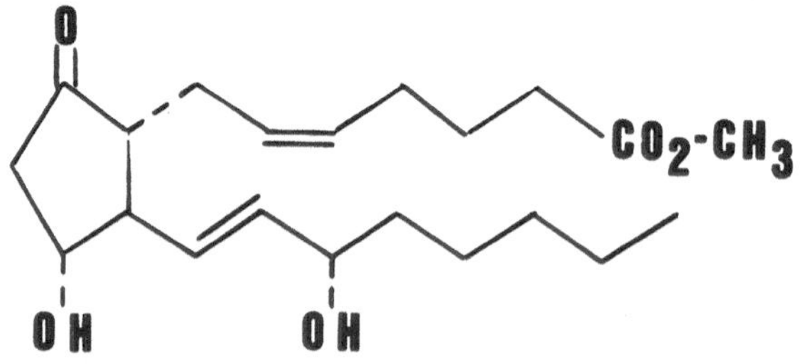

Fig. 1. Structure of $PGE_2$ methyl ester.

15-METHYL ANALOGUES OF PGF$_{2\alpha}$ AND PGE$_2$

15-Methyl-prostaglandins are obtained by incorporation of a methyl group in the 15-position of the parent prostaglandin E$_2$ or F$_{2\alpha}$. This results in the avoidance of C$_{15}$-dehydrogenation, which is the first step in the metabolic inactivation of natural prostaglandins. In addition to this, esterification of the carboxyl function with an additional methyl group may have been performed (Fig. 2).

Characteristic of the 15-methyl derivatives, when compared with the natural prostaglandins, is their increased potency and prolonged duration of action in vivo. Besides, unlike PGE$_2$ and PGF$_{2\alpha}$, intramuscular injection of one of these analogues does not cause local irritation. However, they are not more specifically uterotonic and their systemic administration frequently causes side-effects.

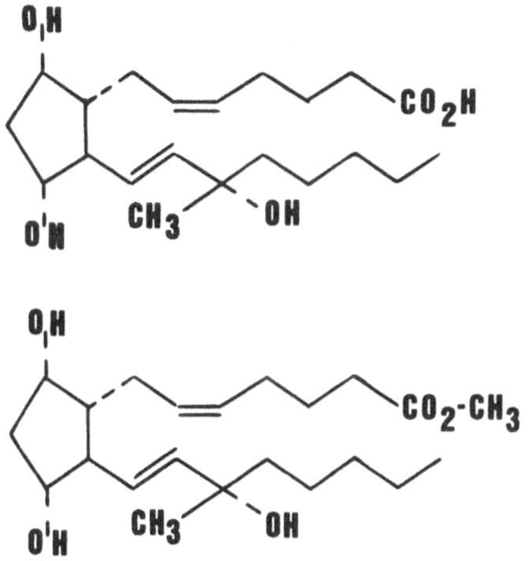

Fig. 2. Structure of 15(S),15-methyl-PGF$_{2\alpha}$ (free acid; top) and of 15(S),15-methyl-PGF$_{2\alpha}$ methyl ester (bottom).

## 15(S),15-Methyl-PGE$_2$ methyl ester

The drug was first tested as an abortifacient by Karim and co-workers (4, 5). Depending upon the route of administration, it appeared to be 80–400 times more oxytocic and (except for the intra-amniotic route) its duration of action was three times longer than that of PGE$_2$. The analogue was administered intramuscularly (25–50 $\mu$g every 8 h), intravaginally (50 $\mu$g every 8 h) or intraamniotically (50–100 $\mu$g every 10 h, or a single injection of 200 $\mu$g). Pregnancy was succesfully terminated in all of the 92 subjects treated.

From these and a subsequent study by the Makerere group (6), one may conclude that 15(S),15-methyl-PGE$_2$ methyl ester is an excellent agent for induction of midtrimester abortion, when given intra-amniotically. Instillation by this route of a single dose of 100 $\mu$g of the analogue caused abortion within 24 h in 90% of the women treated, the remaining 10% being terminated promptly following a second intra-amniotic injection of 100 $\mu$g. With this protocol, the mean time to abortion amounted to 16 $\frac{1}{2}$ h; side-effects were limited to a rise in temperature of 1.0–1.5° C in 15% of the subjects and vomiting in 15% as well. Neither diarrhoea nor shivering was observed [6].

Intramuscular injection of 10 $\mu$g of 15(S),15-methyl-PGE$_2$ methyl ester at 2–4 h intervals interrupted pregnancy within 48 h in 95% of the patients (7–11). Loss of blood amounted only exceptionally to more than 300 ml, and there was minimal pain and discomfort. But other side-effects occurred frequently. Nausea, vomiting and diarrhoea (alone or in combination) were recorded in 45–85% of the cases; shivering, and temperature elevation of 1.0° C or more (occasionally to more than 40.0° C), in 70–100%. Such a major degree of intolerance clearly indicates that this analogue is unsuitable for systemic administration in clinical practice. Despite the interesting results obtained following its intra-amniotic injection (4–6), assessment of the drug ceased after 1975.

## 15(R),15-Methyl-PGE$_2$ methyl ester

This compound is 10 times less oxytocic than its 15(S) counterpart. Nevertheless, it was used succesfully by various routes for termination of pregnancy in a small series of cases [5].

## 15(S),15-Methyl-PGF$_{2\alpha}$ (free acid)

This analogue has a uterotonic potency 20–100 times greater than that of PGF$_{2\alpha}$ and is effect on the myometrium is far longer sustained [4, 12]. Given intravenously at the rate of 5 $\mu$g/min the incidence of side-effects is comparable to that of an equipotent infusion (75 $\mu$g/min) of PGF$_{2\alpha}$ [12]. Wiqvist et al. [13] studied the effects of 1–5 mg 15(S),15-methyl PGF$_{2\alpha}$ instilled intra-amniotically. Uterine activity reached its maximum after 4–9 hours and was maintained at this level throughout the 24-h observation period, or until abortion. A single dose of 1.0, 2.5 or 5.0 mg of the drug terminated pregnancy in 46, 98 and 95% of patients in mean times of 20 h 6 min, 18 h 48 min and 18 h 36 min, respectively. The authors felt that 2.5 mg of the analogue was the optimal dose for 'single-shot' administration by the intra-amniotic route. It was more efficacious and caused fewer side-effects (mean of 1.5 episodes of vomiting per patient) than single doses of 40 mg PGF$_{2\alpha}$ (76% success; mean time to abortion of 18 h 30 min; 3.3 episodes of vomiting) or doses of 25 mg PGF$_{2\alpha}$ repeated after 24 h (97% success; mean time 28 h; 2.0 episodes of emesis). In contra-distinction to the Swedish investigators, Karim and Sivas-amboo [14] reported a success rate of over 90% following an injection of a single dose of 1.0 mg 15(S),15-methyl-PGF$_{2\alpha}$. They felt, as did Krishna et al. [15], that the intra-amniotic instillation of 2.5 mg 15(S),15-methyl-PGF$_{2\alpha}$ caused a prohibitive incidence of gastro-intestinal side effects (Table 1). A WHO multicentre study [16] compared the effects of the intra-amniotic instillation of 2.5 mg of the analogue with that of either 40 or 50 mg PGF$_{2\alpha}$ given by the same route. A higher success rate was obtained with the 15-methyl derivative (92.8–95.6% of subjects aborted within 48 h vs. 81.7–86.6%). Induction-abortion intervals (18–20 h) and rates of complete abortion (51–55%) were similar for both compounds. Although the incidence of heavy bleeding ($\geq$ 500 ml) was less (1.2–2.3 vs. 3.1–3.8%) in patients treated with 15(S),15-methyl-PGF$_{2\alpha}$ and that of cervical injury identical (2.9%), the frequency of vomiting (1.7–2.1 vs. 1.3–1.5 episodes per patient) and diarrhoea (1.2–1.3 vs. 0.4–0.5 episodes) was significantly higher following administration of the analogue. Similar results were reported by Tejuja et al. [17].

The Karolinska group [18] also studied the abortifacient activity of 15(S),15-methyl-PGF$_{2\alpha}$, when given extra-amniotically. The most effective preparation consisted in a mixture of the analogue in Hyskon® (Dextran 70, 32%). A single dose of 500–850 $\mu$g of the prostaglandin in Hyskon® interrupted pregnancy in 84% of the subjects treated within 36 h. The mean time to abortion was 13 h 36 min.

Other studies performed later [15, 19] showed that the extra-amniotic administration of a single dose of 920 $\mu$g 15(S),15-methyl®-PGF$_{2\alpha}$ in Hyskon® was as effective as that of multiple doses of 750 $\mu$g PGF$_{2\alpha}$ via the same route. The time to abortion was shorter but emesis and diarrhoea occurred with a slightly higher frequency (Table 2). MacKenzie and Embrey [20] compared the effects of a single extra-amniotic instillation of 1 mg 15(S),15-methyl-PGF$_{2\alpha}$ suspended in viscous medium (either 4 ml Hyskon® or 8 ml of a gel of Tylose MH 300®, Hoechst, i.e. methyl hydroxyethyl cellulose) to those of 0.5 mg of the analogue in non-viscous medium, the latter injection being repeated after 12 h. The success rate (80% of patients aborted within 24 h) was identical and the mean induction–abortion intervals (16.7–18.1 h, $\pm$ 2.0 h) were very similar in the three groups. However, gastro-intestinal side-effects (vomiting in 50%, diarrhoea in 32.5%) were more frequent in the patients treated with the 1 mg dose in viscous medium. Finally, Tejuja et al. [17] reported on the extra-amniotic injection of 1 mg 15 (S),15-methyl-PGF$_{2\alpha}$ in Hyskon® performed in 1569 cases at 10–20 weeks gestation. Abortion was effected within 36 h in 78.1% of the subjects, in a mean time of 14.8 h. Vomiting was observed in 36.5% and diarrhoea in 33.7% of the women, these rates not being markedly different from those seen by the same investigators

*Table 1* Comparison of $PGF_{2\alpha}$ and 15(S),15-methyl-$PGF_{2\alpha}$ given by the intra-amniotic route for induction of midtrimester abortion

| Compound | Number of patients | Dose (mg) | Success rate (%) | Mean induction-abortion interval (h) | Diarrhoea (mean number of episodes per patient) | Vomiting (mean number of episodes per patient) |
|---|---|---|---|---|---|---|
| $PGF_{2\alpha}$ | 93 | 25 +25 6 hours later | 90 | 22 9 | 0 5 | 1 3 |
| $PGF_{2\alpha}$ | 42 | 40 | 97 | 24 4 | 0 6 | 1 2 |
| $PGF_{2\alpha}$ | 50 | 50 | 100 | 18 9 | 0 2 | 0 8 |
| 15-me-$PGF_{2\alpha}$ | 91 | 2 5 | 100 | 20 3 | 1 8 | 2 1 |

Data from Krishna et al 1978 [15]

*Table 2* Comparison of $PGF_{2\alpha}$ and 15(S),15-methyl-$PGF_{2\alpha}$ given by the extra-amniotic route for induction of midtrimester abortion

| Compound | Number of patients | Dose ($\mu$g) | Success rate (%) | Mean induction-abortion interval (h) | Diarrhoea (mean number of episodes per patient) | Vomiting (mean number of episodes per patient) |
|---|---|---|---|---|---|---|
| $PGF_{2\alpha}$ | 82 | 750 every 2 for 36 h | 78 | 29 1 | 0 4 | 0 8 |
| 15-me-$PGF_{2\alpha}$ | 102 | 920 in Hyskon® gel | 77 | 16 9 | 1 1 | 1 2 |

Data from Krishna et al 1978 [15]

after intra-amniotic instillation of either 50 mg $PGF_{2\alpha}$ or 2.5 mg 15(S),15-methyl-$PGF_{2\alpha}$.

Numerous studies on the intramuscular administration of the analogue for induction of abortion have been published [9, 15, 18, 21–27]. Briefly summarized, injection of 250–750 $\mu$g 15(S),15-methyl-$PGF_{2\alpha}$ every 2 or 3 h caused abortion in 90–100% of the cases in mean times ranging mostly from $13\frac{1}{2}$ to $16\frac{1}{2}$ h. Vomiting was noted in 65–90% of the subjects, and diarrhoea in 53–95%. Temperature elevation of more than 1° C occurred in 15%, but there was no shivering and very little uterine pain. Many feel that the incidence of gastro-intestinal side-effects encountered when 15(S),15-methyl-$PGF_{2\alpha}$ is given intramuscularly is too high — in spite of anti-emetics and anti-diarrhoeics — to recommend this modality of abortion for routine clinical use. Gréen and Bygdeman [28] suggested that the very high plasma levels of the drug measured 20–40 min after intramuscular injection of the analogue and the thereby ensuing stimulation of the gastro-intestinal tract could be avoided by adding 5 $\mu$g epinephrine to the drug before injection. To the best of my knowledge, this suggestion has not been clinically tested.

### 15(S),15-Methyl-$PGF_{2\alpha}$ methyl ester

Vaginal administration of this analogue has been extensively studied. Multicentre studies [15, 29] showed that the vaginal administration every 3 h of a suppository containing 1.5 mg 15(S),15-methyl-$PGF_{2\alpha}$ methyl ester in a mixture of mono-, di- and triglycerides interrupted midtrimester pregnancy within 30 h in 92–98% of the cases. Emesis was noted in up to 67% and diarrhoea in up to 70% of the patients. The incidence of diarrhoea was however much lower in gravidae [15], pre-medicated with diphenoxylate (mean: 1.3 episodes) than in those [29] who were not (mean: 2.8). A temperature of 38° C or more was recorded in 12% of the cases.

When a different vehicle (Witepsol E-76®, Nitro-Nobel AG, Witten, Germany) was used, the release of 15 (S),15-methyl-$PGF_{2\alpha}$ methyl ester from the vaginal suppository was slower. A single such suppository, containing 3.0 mg of the active compound, effected abortion within 24 h in 92% of the subjects, in a mean time of less than 13 h, according to some investigators [30]. Allegedly, due to lesser variations in the plasma concentration of the analogue, side-effects were not as frequent (vomiting: 60% of the case, mean: 1.7 episodes per patient; diarrhoea: 40%, 0.7 episodes) as with the other type of suppository. However, less favourable results, both in terms of efficacy and of tolerance, were reported by Mandelin and Kajanoja [31] after use of these Witepsol E-76® suppositories. In the latter series, only 78% of the patients had aborted within 24 h. The mean time to abortion amounted to 17.9 h. Vomiting was noted in 84% of the cases (mean: 3.2 episodes per subject) and diarrhoea in 66% (mean: 2.5 episodes).

The use of polysiloxane (Silastic®) rings impregnated with 15(S),15-methyl-PGF$_{2\alpha}$ methyl ester and inserted into the vagina for induction of abortion has also been described. The ring is easy to insert and to remove, making it possible to interrupt further release of the drug in case of marked intolerance. Such a device was initially thought to provide a slow and sustained release of the drug. Clinical trials (32–35) using 0.25, 0.5 and 1.0% concentrations of 15 (S),15-methyl-PGF$_{2\alpha}$ methyl ester, containing 10 mg of the drug in each device, have been carried out. Devices of various weights, surface areas and thickness were used. Serial plasma levels of the analogue were determined by some of the investigators [32, 33, 35]). All devices were effective, pregnancy being terminated in 90–100% of subjects treated. Mean induction–abortion intervals amounted to approximately 16–17 h with the 0.25 and 0.5% devices and to 10–11 hours with the 1.0% device. However, absorption of 15 (S),15-methyl-PGF$_{2\alpha}$ methyl ester from the tested polysiloxane rings was extremely variable. The rate of absorption was dependent upon the characteristics of the device (i.e. concentration, surface area, thickness) and the local conditions prevailing in the vagina (presence of blood, amniotic fluid, discharge, etc.). It ensued that side-effects, mainly consisting in vomiting and diarrhoea, were very frequent even in those patients premedicated with prochlorperazine and diphenoxylate hydrochloride. Lauersen and Wilson [36] also reported on the use of a Silastic® ring impregnated with 5 mg of the analogue, in a concentration of 0.5%. The latter device had a markedly lower abortifacient efficacy (56% success). Finally, it should be noted that approximately 10% of the patients in the various series expelled the device prematurely on at least one occassion before abortion and had it reinserted.

### *2a,2b-Dihomo-15(S),15-methyl-PGF$_{2\alpha}$ methyl ester*

Karim [37] reported on the extra-amniotic administration of a single dose of 1 mg of this analogue to a group of 316 women in the late first and early second trimester of pregnancy. Abortion was thus effected in 270 (85.4%) patients of whom 260 (82.3%) aborted within 24 h. All remaining patients given a second dose aborted within the next 24 h. Side-effects with this analogue were less frequent than with 15(S),15-methyl-PGF$_{2\alpha}$. According to the same author [38], 2a,2b-dihomo-15(S),15-methyl-PGF$_{2\alpha}$ methyl ester has since been administered for termination of late first trimester and early second trimester pregnancy to more than 1200 women in Singapore. Results have confirmed the findings of the original study.

16,16-DIMETHYL-PROSTAGLANDINS

These compounds are synthesized by replacing each of the hydrogen atoms attached to $C_{16}$ by a methyl group (Fig. 3). Like the foregoing group, they are not substrates for the enzyme 15-0H-prostaglandin-dehydrogenase. In addition to properties resulting from their slower metabolism, which they share with the 15-methyl-prostaglandins, they display a greater selectivity for the uterus.

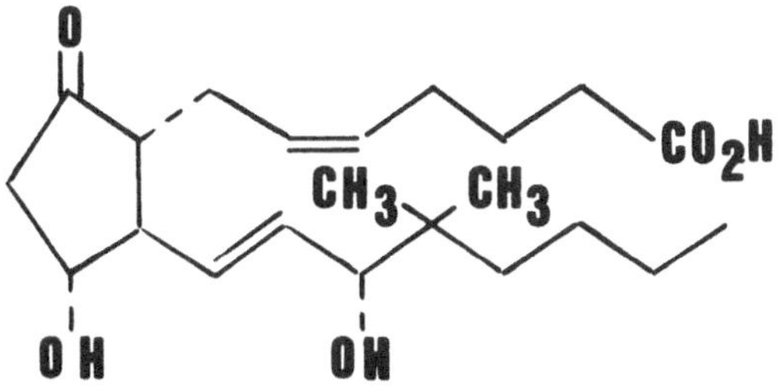

Fig. 3. Structure of 16,16-dimethyl-PGE$_2$.

*16,16-Dimethyl-PGE$_2$ (free acid)*

Martin et al. [39] administered a 400–1200 $\mu$g 16,16-dimethyl-PGE$_2$ vaginal suppository every 2–3 h to 30 women at 13–20 weeks gestation. All but one of the patients aborted within 30 h, in a mean time of 16.8 h ($\pm$ 6.9 h S.D.). Gastro-intestinal side-effects were minimal: 19 of the 30 subjects had no intolerance at all. The overall incidence was 0.7 episode of emesis and 0.3 episode of diarrhoea per patient. Neither anti-emetics nor anti-diarrhoeics were required. There was a slight (less than 1° C) elevation of the temperature in 5 patients; shivering was not noted. Recently [40], a case of corporeal rupture of the uterus was reported in a primigravida at 12 weeks gestation given 9 doses of 1 mg 16,16-dimethyl-PGE$_{2\alpha}$ at 3-h intervals.

The oral administration of this analogue is mentioned in the following section.

*16,16-Dimethyl-PGE$_2$ methyl ester*

Karim and Amy [41] administered 16,16-dimethyl-PGE$_2$ methyl ester by a variety of routes to 23 patients in the second trimester of pregnancy. Vomiting, diarrhoea, pyrexia and shivering were frequently associated with the use of the oral, intravenous and intramuscular routes. Intra-amniotic instillation of 16,16-dimethyl-PGE$_2$ methyl ester caused no side-effects but it required as much as 800 $\mu$g (i.e. 32 times the effective intravenous dose of 25 $\mu$g) in order to accomplish less than adequate uterine stimulation. Of the methods of administration explored, the intravenous injection of one or more doses of 25 $\mu$g had the highest efficacy, but the latter amounted to only 66%. The vaginal route was not assayed in this study. In view of the drawbacks mentioned, the authors felt that the analogue was ill-suited for the induction of abortion. Karim and co-workers [42] were able to terminate 12 out of 20 midtrimester pregnancies by the oral administration of 100 $\mu$g 16,16-dimethyl-PGE$_2$ (free acid or methyl ester) at 2-h intervals. The relatively high incidence of gastro-intestinal side-effects was seen as a limitation to the oral use of these analogues for the purpose of inducing abortion.

## 16,16-Dimethyl-PGE$_2$ p-benzaldehyde-semicarbazone ester

Karim and Ratnam [43] administered vaginally 750 $\mu$g of this analogue in glycerine base suppositories every 4 h to 54 patients in the late first trimester or in the second trimester of pregnancy. Fifty (92.5%) aborted within 36 h. The mean time to abortion amounted to 18.7 h. Side-effects were very mild and consisted of vomiting in 5 patients, diarrhoea in 3 patients and transient pyrexia (38.3° C) in 2. 16,16-Dimethyl-PGE$_2$ p-benzaldehyde-semicarbazone ester given intramuscularly is also effective for interrupting second trimester pregnancy [44]. Doses of 300 $\mu$g, given every 5 h to 36 subjects at 14–22 weeks gestation effected abortion in all in a mean time of 13.4 h (range 2–32 h). Side-effects consisted in vomiting (20% of the cases), diarrhoea (6%) and pyrexia (15%).

## 16,16-Dimethyl-trans-$\Delta^2$-PGE$_1$ methyl ester

Embrey (personal communication, 1980) used this analogue (code name: ONO 802) in 14 patients in the second trimester of pregnancy. The drug was incorporated in a special vehicle and administered intra-vaginally under the from of a suppository. A single dose of 2.5 mg of the active compound effected abortion in 12 of the 14 women (86%) within 24 h. Vomiting was noted in four subjects (29%) and diarrhoea in three (21%).

## 16-PHENOXY-ω-17,18,19,20-TETRANOR-PGE$_2$-METHYLSULPHONAMIDE (SULPROSTONE)

Supprostone is an elaborate, multi-substituted analogue of PGE$_2$ (Fig. 4). Like the 15-methyl- and the 16,16-dimethyl-prostaglandins, it is not a substrate for 15-OH-prostaglandin-dehydrogenase. A fascinating account of the research that led to the synthesis of the analogue can be found in a paper by Hess et al. [45]. It is generally believed to be the prostaglandin with the most

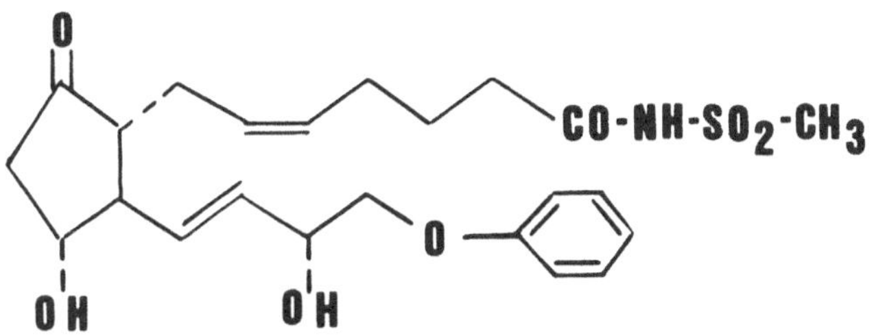

Fig. 4. Structure of 16-phenoxy-ω-17,18,19,20-tetranor-PGE$_2$-methylsulphonamide (sulprostone).

selective uterine stimulant properties available today.

Sulprostone has been administered intra- and extra-amniotically, vaginally, intramuscularly and by intravenous infusion. The latter two methods are as innocuous and as effective as any regimen discussed so far, and, besides, they have the advantage of being technically within the reach of every medical unit.

Schmidt-Gollwitzer [46] intravenously infused 1000 μg sulprostone over 10 h to 184 patients with an intact first or second trimester pregnancy. Abortion occurred in 85.3% of the cases, in a mean time of 12.4 ± 5 h. Nausea and vomiting was observed in 13% of the women and seldom required treatment. The same group of investigators [47] reported that the success rate could be driven up to 100% when patients, having not aborted within 20 h of the start of the first infusion, received a second intravenous infusion of 2000 μg sulprostone administered over 10 h. The mean time to abortion, in this group, was 13.2 h. Side-effects were minor in nature and consisted mainly of uterine pain, nausea and rare episodes of vomiting. Interestingly, no increase in the frequency of side-effects was observed during infusion of this higher dosage. Rizk et al. [48] studied three regimens of intravenous infusion in small groups of gravidae (1000 μg over 4–7 h; 1500 μg over 6 h; 2000 μg over 4 h) and found that 1500 μg infused over 6 h combined a high efficacy (all 7 patients aborted within 24 h) with an acceptable incidence of gastro-intestinal side-effects (mean: 1.3 episodes per patient). The latter authors [48] also studied the abortifacient efficacy of sulprostone given intramuscularly. Injections every 4 h of 500 μg for a maximum of six doses or injections every 6 h of the same amount for a maximum of four doses (the latter schedule used mainly in cases of death in utero) caused 16 out of the 18 women treated to abort within 24 h (mean time to abortion: 11.9 h). Side-effects were limited to minimal gastro-intestinal intolerance (mean: 1.3 episodes per patient), mild uterine cramps and some irritation at the site of injection. Gethmann et al. [49] reported excellent results following injection every 6 h of 1000 μg sulprostone to 40 gravidae at 7–18 weeks gestation. Abortion occurred in 38 of them (95%) in

3–26 h (mean: $11\frac{1}{2}$ h). Vomiting was noted in 7.5%, transient pyrexia and dyspnoea each in 2.5% of the subjects.

Karim [50] compared three different regimens of intramuscular administration of sulprostone (0.5 mg every 4 h; 1.0 mg every 8 h; 1.0 mg every 6 h) in 313 women at 13–24 weeks gestation. Very similar results were recorded in each of the three groups of patients. Pregnancy was successfully interrupted within 36 h in 90–91.5% of the women in each group, in mean times of 17.6–17.9 h (range: $2\frac{1}{4}$–36 h) and at the cost of an acceptable incidence of side-effects (vomiting in 30–39% of the subjects, mean: 0.68–0.78 episode; diarrhoea in 13.5–22.5%, mean 0.23–0.52 episode; shivering in 6.25–13.5%). Three subjects bled more than 500 ml; only one of them required a transfusion. Neither bronchospasm nor any cardiovascular effect was noted. Patients did not complain of pain at the injection sites.

Van den Bergh and Haspels [51] studied the efficacy of several regimens of intra-amniotic administration of sulprostone (1 mg; 2 mg; 3 mg; 3 mg + 2.75 g calcium gluconate; 2 mg + intramuscular oxytocin). Despite the authors' statement, the data reported do not appear to substantiate the greater efficacy of sulprostone when combined with calcium gluconate. With the latter treatment, 87% of the women had aborted within 30 h and 100% within 36 h; but from the information available, it can be calculated that 86.3% of women given 3 mg sulprostone (without calcium gluconate) had aborted within 30 h. (The cumulative abortion rate at 36 hours can not be calculated because of incompleteness of the data.)

Kunz et al. [52] used sulprostone by the extra-amniotic route in 121 gravidae in the first or the second trimester of pregnancy. The administration every hour of 14.29 μg for a total of seven doses (total dose: 100 μg) was more effective (82 and 88% aborted within 24 and 48 h, respectively; induction–abortion interval of 11 h) than the bolus injection of either 50 or 100 μg of the drug. Ulbrich and Bartels [53], reviewing clinical results of several investigators with the extra-amniotic instillation of 25 + 50 μg sulprostone, noted that the cumulative abortion rates at 24 h varied (for similar patient populations) between 60 and 95%, depending on the investigators. They felt that the differences observed were related to the technique of instillation of the analogue, high fundal injection allegedly giving optimal results. Overall, 29% of the subjects had side-effects, generally of very mild intensity.

CONCLUDING REMARKS

The better analogues (Table 3) are more potent and have a longer duration of action than the natural prostaglandin from which they derive. They are also

*Table 3.* Best analogues available in 1980.

a) 2a,2b-dihomo-15(S),15-methyl-PGF$_{2\alpha}$ methyl ester
b) 16,16-dimethyl-PGE$_2$
c) 16,16-dimethyl-PGE$_2$ p-benzaldehyde-semicarbazone ester
d) sulprostone

more specifically uterotonic and may therefore be administered systemically. This requires no particular skills and it eleminates the drawbacks inherent in intra-uterine instillation, in particular by the intra-amniotic route (Table 4). This by no means implies that the use of prostaglandin analogues for in-duction of midtrimester abortion is completely devoid of complications. Overstimulation of the myometrium, following delay in cervical dilatation, will lead to overstretching and tearing of the isthmus, just as it may after use of hypertonic solutions or natural prostaglandins. Delayed post-abortal bleed-ing and shock, following administration of a synthetic prostaglandin, has accounted for at least two maternal deaths [17]. However, with proper

*Table 4.* Advantages of systemic administration.

a) Simple: no expertise required
b) Non invasive: no risk of sepsis
c) Can be used at any stage of gestation
       in patients with ruptured membranes
       in patients with vaginal bleeding
d) The drug acts on the myometrium *and* on the cervix
e) Maintenance of oxytocic effect after expulsion of
       conceptus → decreased risk of haemorrhage

management (Table 5) and by avoiding the intra-amniotic route, whenever possible, this and other complications should become less frequent. Further progress in the field of pharmacological induction of abortion will require much more accurate and more complete reporting of data [54] than has

*Table 5.* Termination of pregnancy with prostaglandins.

Prevention of complications

a) Two-step procedure: 1. Pre-induction ripening of the cervix
                     2. Induction of abortion
b) Avoid overdosage
c) Avoid intra-amniotic route: 1. PG can exert only little ripening
                           effect on the cervix
                      2. Cessation of uterine stimulation
                       after rupture of the membranes
d) Pelvic examination every 4–6 h: thinning of the isthmus?
e) Explore uterine cavity and examine genital tract after every abortion

frequently been the caes so far The majority of papers relating to the use of sulprostone in particular have been of a very poor quality Editors of medical journals and of proceedings of symposia share the responsibility for this matter with the authors

ACKNOWLEDGEMENT

The author is very much indebted to Mrs Bea Pion for expert secretarial assistance

REFERENCES

1 Gillespie A, Beazley JM and Van Dorp DA The use of an 'unnnatural prostaglandin in the termination of pregnancy J Obstet Gynaecol Br Commonw 78 301–304, 1971

2 Sharp DS and Burslem RW The termination of pregnancy by intravenous infusion of a synthetic prostaglandin $F_{2\alpha}$ analogue J Obstet Gynaecol Br Commonw 80 138–141, 1973

3 Karim SMM and Amy JJ Termination of pregnancy with prostaglandin $E_2$ methyl ester Prostaglandins 7 293–302, 1974

4 Karim SMM and Sharma SD Termination of second trimester pregnancy with 15 methyl analogues of prostaglandins $E_2$ and $F_{2\alpha}$ J Obstet Gynaecol Br Commonw 79 737–743, 1972

5 Karim SMM, Sharma SD, Filshie GM, Salmon JA and Adaikan Ganesan P Termination of pregnancy with prostaglandin analogs Adv Biosci 9 811–830, 1973

6 Amy JJ, Karim SMM and Sivasamboo R Intra-amniotic administration of prostaglandin 15(S),15-methyl-$E_2$-methyl ester for termination of pregnancy J Obstet Gynaecol Br Commonw 80 1017–1020, 1973

7 Ballard CA and Quilligan EJ Midtrimester abortion with intramuscular injection of 15-methyl prostaglandin $E_2$ Contraception 9 523–529, 1974

8 Brenner WE, Dingfelder JR and Staurovsky LG The efficacy and safety of intra-muscularly administered 15(S),15 methyl prostaglandin $E_2$ ester for induction of artificial abortion Am J Obstet Gynecol 123 19–31, 1975

9 Gutknecht GD and Southern EM The termination of human pregnancy with prostaglandin analogs J Reprod Med 15 93–96, 1975

10 Laursen NH, Secher NJ and Wilson KH Mid-trimester abortion induced by serial intramuscular injections of 15(S),15-methyl-prostaglandin $E_2$ methyl ester Am J Obstet Gynecol 123 665–670, 1975

11 Stubblefield PG, Naftolin F, Lee EY, Frigoletto FD and Ryan KJ Combination therapy for midtrimester abortion Laminaria and analogues of prostaglandins Contraception 13 723–729, 1976

12 Wiqvist N, Beguin F, Bygdeman M and Toppozada M Recent aspects on systemic administration of prostaglandin In The Prostaglandins — Clinical Applications in Human Reproduction, Southern EM (ed), pp 295–306, Futura, Mount Kisco, 1972

13 Wiqvist N, Bygdeman M and Toppozada M Intra-amniotic prostaglandin administration — a challenge to the currently used methods for induction of midtrimester abortion Contraception 8 113–131, 1973

14 Karim SMM and Sivasamboo R Termination of second trimester pregnancy with intra-amniotic 15(S) 15-methyl-prostaglandin $F_{2\alpha}$ A two dose schedule study Prostaglandins 9 487–494, 1975

15  Krishna U, Ganguli AC, Mandlekar AV and Purandare VN  Administration of prostaglandins by various routes for induction of abortion  merits and demerits  *Prostaglandins* 15 685–693, 1978

16  WHO Task Force on the Use of Prostaglandins for the Regulation of Fertility  Prostaglandins and abortion, III  Comparison of single intra-amniotic injections of 15-methyl-prostaglandin $F_{2\alpha}$ and prostaglandin $F_{2\alpha}$ for termination of second trimester pregnancy  an international multicentric study  *Am J Obstet Gyneacol* 129  601–606, 1977

17  Tejuja S, Choudhury SD and Manchanda PK  Use of intra- and extra-amniotic prostaglandins for the termination of pregnancies — report of multicentric trial in India  *Contraception* 18  641–652, 1978

18  Bygdeman M and Wiqvist N, Induction of abortion by different prostaglandin analogues  *Acta Obstet Gynecol Scand Suppl* 37  67–72, 1975

19  WHO Task Force on the Use of Prostaglandins for the Regulation of Fertility  Prostaglandins and abortion, II  Single extra-amniotic administration of 0 92 mg of 15-methyl-prostaglandin $F_{2\alpha}$ in Hyskon for termination of pregnancies in weeks 10 to 20 of gestation  an international multicentric study  *Am J Obstet Gynecol* 129  593–596, 1977

20  MacKenzie IZ and Embrey MP  Extra-amniotic 15(S)-15 methyl $PGF_{2\alpha}$ to induce abortion  a study of three administration schedules  *Prostaglandins* 12  443–453, 1976

21  Bolognese RJ and Corson SL  Termination of late first-trimester and early second-trimester gestations with intramuscular 15(S),15-methyl-prostaglandin $F_{2\alpha}$  *J Reprod Med* 16  81–84, 1976

22  Gruber W, Brenner WE, Staurovsky LG, Dingfelder JR and Wells JS  Evaluation of intramuscular 15(S),15-methyl-prostaglandin $F_{2\alpha}$ tromethamine salt for induction of abortion, medications to attenuate side effects, and intracervical laminaria tents  *Fertil Steril* 27 1009–1023, 1976

23  Henriques ES, Etkin RH, Lee JD and Schwartz DP  Intramuscular prostaglandin 15(S),15-methyl-$PGF_{2\alpha}$ (THAM) in midtrimester abortion  *Prostaglandins* 13  183–191, 1977

24  Slaughter L and Ballard CA  Midtrimester abortion with intramuscular injection of 15-methyl-prostaglandin $F_{2\alpha}$  *Contraception* 11  533–540, 1975

25  Lauersen NH and Wilson KH  Mid-trimester abortion induced by serial intramuscular injections of 15(S),15-methyl-prostaglandin $F_{2\alpha}$  *Am J Obstet gynecol* 121  273–276, 1975

26  Lange AP and Secher NJ  Midtrimester and missed abortion treated with intramuscular 15(S)15-methyl $PGF_{2\alpha}$  *Prostaglandins* 14  389–395, 1977

27  WHO Task Force on the Use of Prostaglandins for the Regulation of Fertility  Prostaglandins and abortion, I  Intramuscular administration of 15-methyl prostaglandin $F_{2\alpha}$ for induction of abortion in weeks 10 to 20 of pregnancy  *Am J Obstet Gynecol* 129  597–600, 1977

28  Green K and Bygdeman M  Plasma levels of 15(S),15-methyl $PGF_{2\alpha}$ following administration via various routes for induction of abortion  *Prostaglandins* 14  1013–1023, 1977

29  Bygdeman M, Devi PK, Grech ES, Haspels AA, Nyberg R, Purandare VN and Rowe P  Repeated vaginal administration of 15-methyl-$PGF_{2\alpha}$ methyl-ester for termination of pregnancy in the 13th–20th week of gestation  *Contraception* 16  175–181, 1977

30  Bygdeman M, Ganguli A, Kinoshita K, Lundstrom V, Green K and Bergstrom S  Development of a vaginal suppository suitable for single administration for interruption of second trimester pregnancy  *Contraception* 15  129–141, 1977

31  Mandelin M and Kajanoja P  Induction of second trimester abortion  comparison between vaginal 15-methyl-$PGF_{2\alpha}$ methyl ester and intra-amniotic $PGF_{2\alpha}$  *Prostaglandins* 16 995–1001, 1978

32  Lauersen NH and Wilson KH  The abortifacient effectiveness and plasma prostaglandin concentrations with 15(S)-15-methyl prostaglandin $F_{2\alpha}$ methyl ester containing vaginal Silastic devices  *Fertil Steril* 27  1366–1373, 1976

33  Bygdeman M, Green K, Lundstrom V, Ramadan M, Fotiou S and Bergstrom S  Induction of abortion by vaginal administration of 15(S),15-methyl prostaglandin $F_{2\alpha}$ methyl ester  A comparison of two delivery systems  *Prostaglandins* 12 Suppl  27–51, 1976

34 Dillon TF, Mootabar H, Phillips LL and Risk A  The efficacy of intravaginal 15 methyl prostaglandin $F_{2\alpha}$ methyl ester in first and second trimester abortion  *Prostaglandins* 12 Suppl 81–98, 1976

35 Hendricks CH, Dingfelder JR and Gruber WS  Clinical observations with a prostaglandin-containing silastic vaginal device for pregnancy termination  *Prostaglandins* 12 Suppl 99–122, 1976

36 Lauersen NH and Wilson KH  The effect of a 10 cm², 0 5% 15-me-PGF$_{2\alpha}$ methyl ester intravaginal silastic device on abortion and plasma prostaglandin concentration  *Prostaglandins* 13  755–762, 1977

37 Karim SMM  Singapore experience with prostaglandins — routine use and recent advances In  *Obstetric and Gynaecological Uses of Prostaglandins*, Karim SMM (ed), pp  127–154 Eurasia Press, Singapore, 1976

38 Karim SMM  Termination of second trimester pregnancy with prostaglandins  In  *Advances in Prostaglandin Research — Practical Applications of Prostaglandins and their Synthesis Inhibitors*, Karim SMM (ed), pp  375–409  MTP Press, Lancaster, 1979

39 Martin JN Jr, Bygdeman M, Ramadan M, Green K, Leader A, Lundstrom V and Wiqvist N  Vaginally administered 16,16-dimethyl-PGE₂ for the induction of midtrimester abortion  *Prostaglandins* 11  123–132, 1976

40 Jerve F, Fylling P and Stenby S  Rupture of the uterus following treatment with 16-16-dimethyl E₂ prostaglandin vagitories  *Prostaglandins* 17  121–123, 1979

41 Karim SMM and Amy JJ  Effect of prostaglandin 16,16-dimethyl E₂ methyl ester on the pregnant human uterus  *Prostaglandins* 4  581–592, 1973

42 Karim SMM, Sivasamboo R and Ratnam SS  Abortifacient action of orally administered 16,16-dimethyl prostaglandin E₂ and its methyl ester  *Prostaglandins* 6  349–354, 1974

43 Karim SMM and Ratnam SS  Termination of pregnancy with vaginal administration of 16,16-dimethyl-prostaglandin E₂ p-benzaldehyde-semicarbazone ester  *Br J Obstet Gynaecol* 84  135–137, 1977

44 Karim SMM and Ratnam SS  Newer aspects of practical applications of prostaglandins in obstetrics and gynaecology  In  *Biochemical Aspects of Prostaglandins and Thromboxanes*, Kharasch N and Fried J (eds), pp  115–132, Academic Press, New York, 1977

45 Hess HJ, Schaaf TK, Bindra JS, Johnson MR and Constantine JW  Structure–activity considerations leading to sulprostone  In  *International Sulprostone Symposium*, Friebel K, Schneider A and Wurfel H (eds), pp  29–37, Schering AG, Berlin, 1979

46 Schmidt-Gollwitzer M, Schussler B, Schmidt-Gollwitzer K, Elger W and Nevinny-Stickel J Termination of pregnancy by intravenous administration of sulprostone, a tissue-selective PGE₂ derivate  *Singapore J Obstet Gynaecol* 9  63–67, 1978

47 Schmidt-Gollwitzer M, Schuessler B, Schmidt-Gollwitzer K and Nevinny-Stickel J  Recommendations for the treatment of induction of abortion with sulprostone  In  *International Sulprostone Symposion*, Friebel K, Schneider A and Wurfel H (eds), 119–126, Schering AG, Berlin, 1979

48 Rizk MA, Sallam AN, Nayel SA, El-Damarawy H and Toppozada MK  Therapeutic abortion with a prostaglandin suitable for systemic use  *Singapore J Obstet Gynaecol* 9 57–62, 1978

49 Gethmann U, Hoppen HO and Oberheuser F  Termination of first and second trimester pregnancy with intramuscular administration of sulprostone, a new prostaglandin analogue, *IRCS Med Sci* 6  423, 1978

50 Karim SMM  Prostaglandins in Obstetrics and Gynaecology  In  *International Sulprostone Symposium*, Friebel K, Schneider A and Wurfel H (eds), pp  7–28, Schering AG, Berlin, 1979

51 Van den Bergh AS and Haspels AA  Termination of second trimester pregnancy with intraamniotic administration of 16-phenoxy-$\omega$-tetranor-PGE₂-methyl-sulfonamide (SHB 286) alone and combined with oxytocin and calcium gluconate  *Contraception* 18 635–639, 1978

52. Kunz J, Kunz-Padrutt M, Bänninger U, Reich P and Keller PJ: Abortinduktion im 1. und 2. Trimenon durch extraamniale Instillation eines Prostaglandin $E_2$-Derivates. *Geburtshilfe Frauenheilkd* 39: 798–808, 1979.

53. Ulbrich I and Bartels H: Clinical results with sulprostone. In: *International Sulprostone Symposium*, Friebel K, Schneider A, Wurfel H (eds), pp. 61–66, Schering AG, Berlin, 1979.

54. Amy JJ, Thiery M, Bygdeman M, Kerenyi TD, Crawford JS and Karim SMM: A suggested set of working definitions and criteria applicable to interruption of pregnancy. *Contraception* 14: 193–197, 1976.

# 13. PROSTAGLANDIN THERAPY FOR SECOND TRIMESTER ABORTION: AN OVERVIEW OF CURRENT STATUS AND RECENT TRENDS

## M.P. EMBREY

Although their introduction as potent abortifacients was widely hailed in the late 1960s, the prostaglandins (PGs) have not yet realised their full potential in fertility regulation and, especially in the termination of early pregnancy, experience has so far fallen short of expectations. However, the prostaglandins have established a role in the termination of second trimester pregnancy. In Britain the method is increasingly popular; approximately 20% of all midtrimester abortions are induced with prostaglandins and in many units prostaglandins are used to the exclusion of other methods. In the United States on the other hand, where experience has been virtually confined to intra-amniotic $PGF_{2\alpha}$, the proportion of prostaglandin abortions is rather less and the respective merits of prostaglandins and the alternative methods, intra-amniotic saline and surgical evacuation are vigorously debated.

### NATURAL PROSTAGLANDINS

The value and limitations of the natural prostaglandins ($PGE_2$ and $PGF_{2\alpha}$) have been reviewed elsewhere (Craft, chapter 11). Their shortcomings as abortifacients are related to their rapid inactivation and the degree of gastro-intestinal irritation produced by systemic absorption. In summary, oral therapy is ineffective, intravenous therapy requires high dosage and causes unacceptable side effects while vaginal administration also results in prominent side effects and is not consistently successful. However, intra-uterine administration by the extra-amniotic or intra-amniotic routes can give generally satisfactory results and both have been extensively used.

A large experience of intra-amniotic $PGF_{2\alpha}$ has shown that, for an acceptable level of efficacy (90 + % abortions in 48 h; mean abortion time 24 h), an injection of 25 mg frequently needs to be repeated (in 24 or 6 h) or the initial dose has to be increased to 40–50 mg and both regimes result in troublesome gastro-intestinal side-effects [1].

Though it has been less frequently used, several trials have shown the effectiveness of intra-amniotic $PGE_2$. The administration of 20 mg or 10 mg repeated in 6 h, gives a high success rate (95% in 24 h) with relatively few side-effects.

*M J N C Keirse et al (eds ), Second Trimester Pregnancy Termination All rights reserved*
*Copyright © 1982 Martinus Nijhoff Publishers, The Hague/Boston/London*

The efficacy of the extra-amniotic method is comparable with that of the intra-amniotic route. Early trials showed that instillation every 2 h of $PGE_2$ 200 $\mu$g or $PGF_{2\alpha}$ 750 $\mu$g, or equivalent amounts by continuous infusion, results in abortion within 48 h in approximately 90% of patients [1]. Later it was demonstrated that the administration of 1.5–3 mg $PGE_2$ in a viscous gel provides a more prolonged effect, limiting the need for frequent or continuous injection, and gives equivalent results. Nowadays this is the method usually employed. Because of the low dosage used the incidence of gastro-intestinal effects is lower with extra-amniotic than with other routes of administration while the theoretical risk of infection has not proved a serious hazard in practice.

Personal views are based on experience of prostaglandins over 10 years in Oxford, where referrals in the second trimester still account for some 15% of the total abortions performed. For several years virtually all these have been prostaglandin terminations and as a routine extra-amniotic $PGE_2$ is still the method most frequently used (Fig. 1).

The preference for $PGE_2$ dates from 1969 [2] when we first observed its greater utero-tonic potency compared with $PGF_{2\alpha}$. Additionally, experience has shown that side-effects are generally less severe with $PGE_2$, which continues to be the preferred natural compound.

We advocated administration of $PGE_2$ by the extra-amniotic route in 1970, noting the comparatively low total dosage required and consequently low level of gastro-intestinal side-effects. Having shown that, if prescribed in a viscous gel, a single injection usually suffices, we subsequently pioneered the

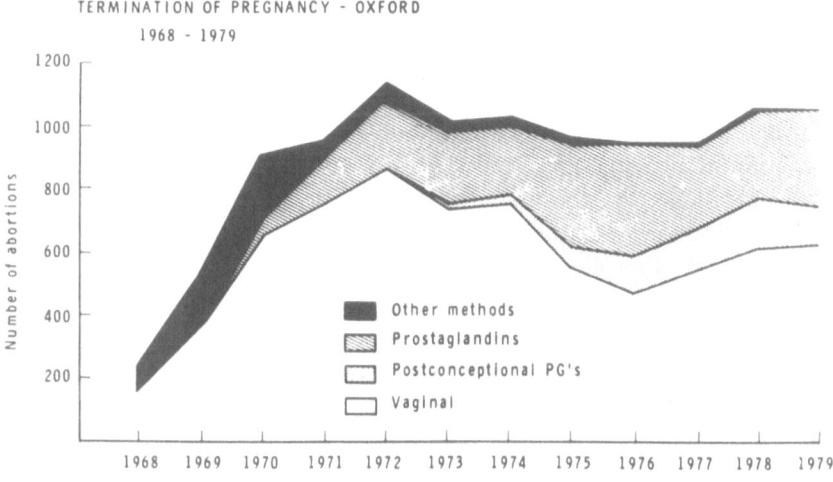

*Fig. 1.* Methods used for termination of pregnancy in Oxford from 1968 to 1979.

$PGE_2$/gel method [3]. Extra-amniotic $PGE_{2\alpha}$ gel continues to be used extensively and intra-amniotic $PGE_2$ to a lesser extent.

To shorten abortion times and increase reliability we routinely use the enhancement effect of oxytocin. In this way, for both extra- and intra-amniotic routes, 95% success within 24 h with low side effects is achieved (Table 1). Intra-amniotic hypertonic solutions to augment prostaglandin activity can cause adverse effects, e.g. coagulopathy, hypernatraemia, and are only used for gestations above 20 weeks to ensure lack of foetal viability.

*Table 1*. Prostaglandin-induced midtrimester abortion (till March 1978).

| | No. of cases | Abortion times (%) | | | Side-effects (%) | | |
|---|---|---|---|---|---|---|---|
| | | % < 12 h | % < 24 h | complete | V* | D* | Nil |
| *Extra-amniotic* | | | | | | | |
| $PGE_2$ 2.5 mg/gel + IV oxytocin at 6 h | 77 | 53.2 | 98.7 | 61.0 | 49.3 | 22.1 | 45.4 |
| *Intra-amniotic* | | | | | | | |
| $PGE_2$ 10 mg + 10 mg at 6 h + IV oxytocin | 68 | 64.7 | 95.6 | 75.0 | 67.6 | 8.8 | 30.9 |

* V, Vomiting; D, Diarrhoea

PROSTAGLANDIN ANALOGUES

Chemists in recent years have sought to overcome the limitations of the natural prostaglandins by the synthesis of analogues which, by resisting metabolic degradation, exhibit enhanced potency and longer action or show greater specificity of action so causing fewer side-effects. To a degree these efforts have been successful and the developments have refocused attention particularly on the potential merits of vaginal administration. However, the clinical trials (reviewed by Amy, chapter 12) have shown that not all the problems have been resolved.

Thus, although the utero-tonic potency of the 15 methyl-derivatives of $PGE_2$ and $PGF_{2\alpha}$ is high, the severity of gastro-intestinal and other side-effects accompanying administration by routes depending on system absorption (e.g. intramuscular, vaginal) limits their clinical applicability.

More selective in action, the 16:16-dimethyl-$PGE_2$ analogue and its p-benzaldehyde semicarbazone ester cause fewer adverse effects, have been shown to be effective by vaginal administration in simple glyceride based pessaries and would have considerable clinical impact, were it not that problems of stability have hampered production[4].

Unfortunately, the same lack of stability characterises other recent PGE derivatives which have been shown to be effective abortifacients although causing relatively few side-effects. One of these, 16-phenoxy-$\omega$-tetranor-

$PGE_2$ (Schering), has given encouraging results by the intramuscular route while 16:16-dimethyl-trans-$\Delta_2$-$PGE_1$ (ONO 802) has shown a welcome combination of efficacy and low side-effects when administered in vaginal pessaries.

In Oxford, interest in vaginal administration has centred principally on its role for early post-conceptional abortion (menstrual induction). However, second trimester terminations have been studied also, although the attraction of a non-invasive method in mid-pregnancy is somewhat offset by the proportion of incomplete abortions requiring evacuation.

Our own work and the reported experience of others have shown us the potential of the vaginal pessary method but equally the disadvantages of the products so far available, namely:

1) The pessaries used, of simple formulation, mostly require repeated administration.
2) The level of side-effects with PGF-derived analogues (e.g. 15-methyl-$PGF_{2\alpha}$) is unacceptably high.
3) Recent more promising PGE-derived analogues (e.g. 16:16-dimethyl-$PGE_2$) lack adequate long-term stability.

It has become increasingly evident to us that an improved delivery vehicle providing stability and sustained release could have considerable potential. Over the past two years, therefore, we have been developing a water swellable, cross-linked, polymer-based pessary (Hydrogel) for sustained release of prostaglandins and PG analogues. Working first with $PGE_2$ in vitro it was shown that relatively constant release over prolonged periods of time could be achieved and, moreover, that the device could be readily 'tailored' to prolong or accelerate release to provide a desired release profile. We are now using a $PGE_2$ polymer pessary for cervical ripening in labour induction[5].

Using a similar device for induction of abortion preliminary clinical studies have so far been undertaken with 16:16-dimethyl-$PGE_2$-parabenzaldehyde-semicarbazone ester (Upjohn), and with 16:16-dimethyl-trans-$\Delta_2$-$PGE_1$ (ONO 802). The two prostaglandin analogues exhibit differing release characterisctics requiring appropriate modification of the pessary. The dose released is the significant factor and in the exploratory stage the amount of analogue incorporated in the pessary varied depending on its release profile. The indications are that dose requirements for the two compounds are similar and exemplified by the recent use of a pessary containing 2.5–3 mg of analogue with a half-life of 8–10 h (Fig. 2).

Clinically both analogues have given promising results, a single pessary resulting in successful abortion within 24 h in nearly 90% of patients with comparatively few gastrointestinal symptoms. The studies are being extended but already in this novel polymer device there is promise of a solitary prostaglandin pessary for reliable induction of abortion with low side-effects (Table 2).

136

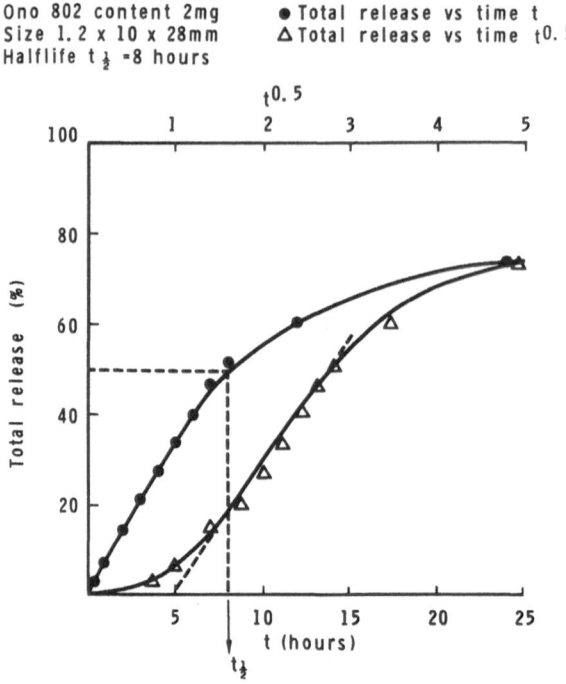

Ono 802 content 2mg
Size 1.2 x 10 x 28mm
Halflife t ½ =8 hours

● Total release vs time t
△ Total release vs time $t^{0.5}$

*Fig. 2.* Release of the prostaglandin analogue ONO 802 from a dry PEO slice into buffer solution (pH 7.4) at 37°C. C.

Apart from the development of better delivery vehicles to facilitate vaginal therapy other developments can be expected too.

Current prostaglandin research aims at developing improved analogues with prolonged effects, greater specificity of action, improved stability and minimal side-effects. One new $PGE_2$ derivative, 9-de-oxo-16:16-dimethyl-9-methylene-$PGE_2$, a potent uterotonic reported to possess increased stability, is already undergoing clinical testing.

Additionally, other new prostaglandin derivatives being studied include at

*Table 2.* Midtrimester abortion induced by PGE analogues in a sustained release polymer vaginal pessary.

| Analogue | No. of cases | Abortion | Complete | Vomiting | Diarrhoea |
|---|---|---|---|---|---|
| 16:16-dimethyl-$PGE_2$-semi-carbazone ester | 28 | 25 (89%) | 21 | 5 | 5 |
| 16:16-dimethyl-trans-$\Delta_2$-$PGE_1$ | 14 | 12 (85%) | 9 | 4 | 3 |

least one with enhanced stability and two with reported luteolytic effects Results in animal studies have been promising, although these compounds have not yet been tested on women The developments are encouraging and it seems likely that new prostaglandin analogues and delivery systems will offer improvement on, and eventually supplant, present day abortion techniques

REFERENCES

1 Embrey MP and Hillier K Prostaglandins in reproduction In *Recent Advances in Obstetrics and Gynaecology*, Stallworthy J and Bourne G (eds), pp 75–104 Churchill-Livingstone, London, 1977
2 Embrey MP The effect of prostaglandins on the human pregnant uterus *J Obstet Gynaecol Br Commonww* 76 783–798, 1969
3 MacKenzie IZ, Hillier K and Embrey MP Singly extra-amniotic injection of prostaglandin $E_2$ in viscous gel to induce mid-trimester abortion *Br med J* 1 240–242, 1975
4 Karim SMM and Ratnam SS Termination of pregnancy with vaginal administration of 16 16-dimethyl-prostaglandin $E_2$ p-benzaldehyde semicarbazone ester *Br J Obstet Gynaecol* 84 135–137, 1977
5 Graham NB, McNeill ME, Zulfigan M and Embrey MP Hydrogels for the controlled release of prostaglandin $E_2$ American Chemical Society Meeting, Houston, *Polymer Reprints* 21 104, 1980

# 14. TERMINATION OF PREGNANCY AFTER INTRAUTERINE FOETAL DEATH

## MARC J.N.C. KEIRSE

Foetal death in utero may occur at any stage of pregnancy. In the first trimester, the termination of such pregnancies poses few problems and is effected by a simple dilatation and vacuum aspiration or curettage. Although in the second trimester the uterus can still be evacuated vaginally by mechanical means, this is by no means as simple as in the first trimester. With advancing gestational age there is increasing difficulty in evacuating foetal bones and skull in addition to the risk of excessive loss of blood.

In a way the termination of such pregnancies at once differs from and resembles that of other second trimester terminations. Although still practised, the time-honoured therapy of procrastination is increasingly being challenged by a greater responsiveness to the emotional needs and wishes of the patient, earlier and better detection of foetal death, improved methods for terminating such pregnancies, etc. In the meantime advances in perinatology have lowered the average gestational age at which foetal death occurs. These advances and changes in nomenclature further obliterate the old distinction between missed abortion and missed labour, and challenge the concept that the management of intrauterine foetal death can be demarcated by gestational dividing lines.

The object of the present chapter is to draw attention to these changes and to examine their implications for the management of intrauterine foetal death after the first trimester of pregnancy.

THE CHANGES AND THEIR EFFECTS

*The trimester threshold, missed abortion and missed labour*

For many years, termination of pregnancy has been greatly influenced by the obstetrical tradition to customarily divide pregnancy into three equal parts known as trimesters. Although that division appears to stand or fall with an accurate definition of weeks of pregnancy, the latter are by no means uniformly defined (Tietze, chapter 1). Yet it was demonstrated elsewhere (Cates and Grimes, chapter 5) how the myth of a trimester threshold may overrule all concepts of gestation as a continuum and determine practices of pregnancy termination. In cases of intrauterine death, the trimester threshold gains some additional complexity in that it is not always clear whether demise or expulsion of the foetus is considered as the cut-off point. Yet the threshold myth (Cates and Grimes, chapter 5) remains fully applicable; even more so, since there is now also an upper limit to be considered. It is still common practice to use the 28th week of pregnancy as a cut-off point between *missed abortion* and *missed labour*. The latter will then result in stillbirth, but so may the former, since missed abortion is not infrequently defined by the time of foetal death instead of foetal expulsion. The 28 weeks tenet has led some [1] to introduce separate recommendations for the management of missed abortion and missed labour. As will be discussed below, the available data indicate that these too may have evolved from the realm of myth and clinical impression rather than from the reality of clinical observations.

The only valid basis for a 28 weeks cut-off point has been the fact that this was also the international criterion for inclusion into perinatal mortality statistics. However, since both WHO and FIGO [2, 3] have redefined the criteria for inclusion in such statistics to a birthweight of 1000 g or more there is no further need for this confusion. In addition, the cut-off point between abortion and birth has now been placed at 500 g [2, 3], which has annihilated the old distinction between missed abortion and missed labour. Whether the case should be labelled as abortion, birth and/or perinatal mortality now depends entirely upon birthweight. This can only be ascertained after termination of pregnancy and is therefore of no value for the choice of management. Obviously these arguments do not reduce gestational age to an irrelevant item in the management of foetal death. By abolishing the threshold myth they reveal that, for practical purposes, gestational age acts as a continuum rather than as a demarcation. This principle will be adhered to and further examined in this presentation.

*The circumstances of intrauterine foetal death*

The circumstances of intrauterine foetal death have changed considerably and in several respects over the past few decades. The average duration of pregnancy at which foetal death occurs has decreased. For instance, if only the more reliable data of stillbirth beyond 28 weeks of gestation are considered, the 1958 British Perinatal Mortality Survey [4] reports that less than half of these occurred below 37 weeks, as compared to the majority of cases in studies of the 1970s [5]. Of all intrauterine foetal deaths that occurred after the 16th week of pregnancy and before the onset of labour in our department during the years 1977–79, 55% occurred before 28 weeks and 91% before 37 weeks. This implies that the interval between foetal demise and the normally expected date of delivery is now very much longer.

Several large studies [6, 7] have shown that labour will begin spontaneously within 2 to 3 weeks after foetal death in over 80% of women. However, there are no means at present to foretell when labour will start, although the interval is to some extent dependent on the cause of foetal death [6]. In consideration of foetal and placental causes, Csapo [8] has related the interval to residual placental endocrine function (Table 1). However, the same study [6] showed that, when foetal death was thought to be due to cord accidents, the interval till delivery took an average of 4.6 days, which is shorter than that in cases of toxaemia (Table 1). Furthermore, in 65 women harbouring a dead foetus for 3 days to 8 weeks, Schulman et al. [9] found progesterone levels within the normal statistical range for gestation averaging approximately 80% of the mean, but no correlation was made with the duration of foetal death. On the other hand, gestational age at the time of foetal death appears to have a distinct influence on the interval till delivery. Although it is not easy to distinguish this influence from that of the aetiology of foetal death, Grandin and Hall [6] showed that the earlier in gestation foetal death occurs the longer the interval till delivery will be (Table 2). This indicates that the present

*Table 1* Relationship between the cause of foetal death and the interval between foetal death and delivery (adapted from Csapo (8) after data from Grandin and Hall (6)

| Cause of foetal death | Estimated residual placental function | No of cases (N = 188) | Average gestational age at foetal death (weeks) | Mean interval between foetal death and delivery (days) |
|---|---|---|---|---|
| Abruption | None or minimal | 58 | 35 | < 2 |
| Toxaemia | Hypofunction | 94 | 35 | 6 8 |
| Rhesus disease | Normal | 36 | 34 | 14 3 |

*Table 2* Relationship between gestational age at the time of foetal death before labour and the interval until delivery (after Grandin and Hall (6), with exclusion of cases of abruptio placentae and cases in which the duration of foetal death before delivery was unknown)

| Gestational age at foetal death (weeks) | Total number of cases | Interval between foetal death and delivery | | | | | |
|---|---|---|---|---|---|---|---|
| | | More than 1 week | | More than 2 weeks | | More than 4 weeks | |
| | | No | % | No | % | No | % |
| <32 | 84 | 31 | 36 9 | 21 | 25 0 | 16 | 19 0 |
| 33–37 | 116 | 27 | 23 3 | 13 | 11 2 | 3 | 2 6 |
| 38–42 | 99 | 18 | 18 2 | 6 | 6 1 | 3 | 3 0 |
| >42 | 8 | 1 | 12 5 | 0 | – | 0 | – |
| Total | 307 | 77 | 25 1 | 40 | 13 0 | 22 | 7 2 |

tendency for foetal death to occur earlier in pregnancy may imply a longer interval to the actual date of delivery as well as to the normally expected date.

Another factor is that the care of pregnancy has changed greatly, particularly in our western world. Pregnancy, or at least a continuing pregnancy, is no longer a fate that befalls women but a cherished option. It implies earlier and more regular antenatal care, a greater awareness of possible complications, the significance of quickening and the absence thereof. Foetal death is therefore more readily suspected and brought to medical attention than used to be the case.

In the past a suspicion of foetal death had to be viewed with caution. Confirmation depended on tests, such as urinary oestrogen or gonadotrophin excretion or radiological signs, which require an appropriate delay after fetal demise in order to be conclusive. Many obstetricians have been rewarded for adopting a cautious, expectant attitude by the birth of a live infant thought to be dead several days or weeks before. Less prudent clinicians, who have terminated such pregnancies on rather flimsy grounds, have delivered live infants that were subsequently lost to hyaline membrane disease. To our knowledge, the last such case was reported as recently as 1979 [10]. At present there can be no excuse for such errors, nor for a substantial delay in arriving at a correct diagnosis. Modern techniques, such as cardiotocography, ultrasound and real-time scanning will occasionally document the time of foetal death and should certainly allow a correct diagnosis to be established with a minimum of delay.

The net result of these combined changes signifies that foetal death now occurs earlier in pregnancy, is more readily suspected and is diagnosed almost as soon as it is suspected. Even if such changes did not influence the interval between foetal demise and the onset of labour, a greater deal of that interval is now spent knowingly carrying a dead foetus and that at a time when the expected end of pregnancy is still a long way off. All of these factors intensify the mental distress and emotional anguish of the patient in carrying a dead foetus as the major problem to be dealt with in cases of intrauterine foetal death.

*The advent of prostaglandins to replace dangerous or ineffective approaches*

In the past this mental distress needed to be carefully balanced against the dangers of rather ineffective measures to actively expel the foetus and the somatic risks of intrauterine retention of a dead foetus. The somatic risks to which a woman with intrauterine retention of a dead foetus is exposed are small. The most serious complication is a disturbance of the blood coagulation mechanisms. There may be a progressive decline in platelets and fibrinogen levels, when the foetus has been dead for three weeks or more, but

Pritchard [11] showed that this is unlikely to result in clinical complications in less than five weeks after foetal death. On the other hand, one may argue that speedy delivery will increase the possibility of discovering the cause of foetal death by chromosome analysis and pathological examination of foetus and placenta [12]. However, this will only apply if the interval can be kept short enough. Hence, from a strictly somatic point of view there is little to be gained by an active management of foetal death. In the past elective attempts at induction have not infrequently turned into iatrogenic nightmares, because of the unreliability and the risks of the available methodology. The older literature contains cases that failed to deliver in spite of repeated attempts over the course of anything up to two years [13]. Oestrogen administration used to be a favourite treatment some 40 years ago, but this needed to be given for several days, was rather ineffective [14] and may most appropriately be described as a method of playing for time [13]. Another approach has been the intra-amniotic injection of hypertonic solutions. This is more dangerous than in intact pregnancies (see Kerenyi, chapter 8) for several reasons, including the frequency of oligohydramnios, difficulties of identifying the uterine cavity, the altered permeability of the foetal membranes [15] and a predisposition of such cases to develop coagulation disorders [11]. Finally, the number of fatalities that has been reported has been sufficient to discourage a wider adoption of the method [13]. Of the many alternatives that have been used in the past, high doses of oxytocin were the most successful [16], but effective doses nearly always led to some degree of water retention [17]. Combining oxytocin therapy with amniotomy could increase the effectiveness and shorten the induction–delivery interval [18] but at the expense of risking intrauterine infection if the method fails. Up to the present decade, many gynaecologists have therefore used intravenous infusion of moderate to high doses of oxytocin for a limited period of time, repeating the process after an adequate period of rest if it did not work. Not surprisingly, instead of diminishing the emotional anguish of the patient, this procedure often added to it, leaving the patient totally exasperated after every failed attempt to induce labour.

At present the above situation has been drastically changed by the introduction of prostaglandins and their analogues. Cumulative experience with these compounds in the management of intrauterine foetal death has grown rapidly since their introduction in 1970 [19] and has proved their high effectiveness in the management of foetal death. The incidence of serious complications has been low and these were often related to inappropriate use or to a combination with other procedures [20] and/or oxytocic drugs [9]. In addition, many studies have shown that there are no significant alterations in the coagulation system with the use of either prostaglandins [21] or their analogues [22].

PROSTAGLANDINS FOR THE MANAGEMENT OF INTRAUTERINE DEATH

The cumulative experience with prostaglandins and their analogues to terminate pregnancy after intrauterine foetal death now includes thousands of cases which cannot appropriately be reviewed in the context of a single chapter. Karim et al. [1] recently reviewed the English literature data and neatly summarized the results of some 50 reports in a series of tables. A general summary of their tables is presented in Table 3. From this table one can to some extent appreciate the heterogeneity of the data that were reviewed and safely confirm the authors' conclusion on the effectiveness of prostaglandins, administered by various routes, for terminating pregnancy after intrauterine foetal death.

In fact, our experience [23, 24] and that of others [1, 9] indicates that such pregnancies can be terminated more readily with prostaglandins than viable pregnancies at corresponding gestational ages. The reason for this phenomenon is not clear. It has been attributed to lower progesterone concentrations [8, 9]. However, Schulman et al. [9] found progesterone levels to be within the normal statistical range for gestation averaging approximately 80% of the mean. Moreover the dose-delivery response in 65 cases did not correlate with progesterone levels [20]. The high 15-hydroxy-prostaglandin dehydrogenase content, the enzyme responsible for inactivation of prostaglandins, of viable placental tissue and foetal membranes [25, 26] has been proffered as another

Table 3. Cumulative experience with natural prostaglandins administered by various routes for termination of pregnancy after intrauterine foetal death (all gestational ages summarized from tabular material of Karim et al. (1)).

| Prostaglandin and route of administration | No. of cases | Successfully treated | | Mean total dose (mg) | | Mean induction-delivery interval (h:min) | |
|---|---|---|---|---|---|---|---|
| | | No. | % | Lowest | Highest | Median | Range[1] |
| Intravenous $PGE_2$[2] | 269 | 255 | 94.8 | 0.58 – | 7.30 | 11:22 | 7:42[3]–17:26 |
| Intravenous $PGF_{2\alpha}$[2] | 174 | 166 | 95.4 | 8.7 – | 52.3 | 9:20 | 7:00–19:15 |
| Extra-amniotic $PGE_2$ | 115 | 112 | 97.4 | 0.45 – | 3.80 | 8.48 | 7:06–17:12 |
| Extra-amniotic $PGF_{2\alpha}$ | 41 | 40 | 97.6 | 3.5 – | 120 | 12:00 | 10:12–15:44 |
| Intra-amniotic $PGF_{2\alpha}$ | 86 | 85 | 98.8 | 5.6 – | 78.3 | 10:50 | 8:22–10:57 |
| Vaginal $PGF_2$[4] | 899 | 872 | 97.0 | 26 – | 90 | 9:30 | 6:18–14:36 |
| Total | 1584 | 1530 | 96.6 | | | | 6:18–19:15 |

[1] The median is based on all mean induction-delivery intervals reported; the range relates only to those means that are based on more than 6 cases.
[2] Infusion rates ranged from 0.5 to 12.0 µg/min for $PGE_2$ and from 2.5 to 200 µg/min for $PGF_{2\alpha}$.
[3] The patients in that study were given simultaneous oxytocin infusion; the next lowest mean is 8:30.
[4] One study (28) that used $PGE_2$ and $PGF_{2\alpha}$ is not included.

possible explanation [23]. However, a similar difference in uterine sensitivity between viable pregnancies and cases of foetal death appears to apply to prostaglandin analogues that are resistant to degradation by 15-hydroxy-prostaglandin dehydrogenase [24, 1].

So far few investigators have taken these observations into account in determining the dose of prostaglandin required [27]. Dose schedules for terminating pregnancy after foetal death have generally been based on those used for second trimester termination of pregnancy, since adequate experience is more easily gathered in this area. Some investigators have used even higher doses than those required to terminate viable pregnancies which has led to uterine overstimulation in several instances, excessively high incidences of side-effects and occasional damage to the uterus or cervix [1]. It cannot be overemphasized that with respect to doses and route of administration of prostaglandins, cases of foetal death need to be considered separately from other terminations of pregnancy.

*Choice of prostaglandin and route of administration*

The ideal therapeutic agent for the management of intrauterine foetal death should be effective, easy to administer and free of hazards or serious side-effects. Provided that some basic principles, such as a five- to tenfold higher potency of $PGE_2$, are adhered to, the choice between the two natural prostaglandins $PGF_{2\alpha}$ and $PGE_2$ appears to depend mainly on availability of the drug and acquired experience of the person administering it. Otherwise the results are rather similar (Table 3), though at present exception should be made for the vaginal and oral routes.

Intravenous infusion of both prostaglandins is far more effective than in other terminations of pregnancy (Craft, chapter 11) and side-effects are mainly encountered when large doses are employed in an attempt to shorten the induction–delivery interval. Nevertheless, in view of their short half-life in the circulation there is a general tendency to resort to local, intrauterine administration of these compounds for termination of pregnancy (Craft, chapter 11).

Administered intra-amniotically these compounds are effective in cases of foetal death but there are major objections to this approach. As discussed above with regard to the use of hypertonic saline, the procedure may be technically difficult, alterations in the membranes need to be considered and there is a potential risk of introducing infection which may be particularly troublesome in the presence of a dead foetus. Hence this approach is not to be recommended and experience with it has been limited [1].

Extra-amniotic administration particularly by continuous infusion or by the rather cumbersome approach of repeated doses is highly effective too.

Bolus doses need to be larger, are likely to produce side-effects and offer no advantage. However, extra-amniotic administration requires some expertise and experience in order to avoid rupture of the membranes, introduction of infection and premature expulsion of the catheter. The latter occurs in a significant proportion of patients and may necessitate administration of intravenous prostaglandins or oxytocin to ensure completion of the procedure [1].

Vaginal administration combines simplicity with ease of administration. Recently, all studies have been concerned with $PGE_2$, although the first report on vaginal administration dealt with both $PGE_2$ and $PGF_{2\alpha}$, in doses of 20 and 50 mg respectively [28]. It should be realized that its effect depends on systemic absorption. Hence, the incidence of gastrointestinal and other side-effects is high. For instance a large multicentre trial of 709 patients reported vomiting in 56%, diarrhoea in 43%, chills and shivering in 22% and pyrexia exceeding 38.1° C in 40% of cases [29]. Fear of infection may well lead to an excessive and unnecessary use of antibiotics in such cases. In addition the procedure is likely to be complicated if rupture of the membranes or bleeding occurs early during treatment since this may interfere with the administration and absorption of subsequent doses.

Oral prostaglandins can only be given in small doses since gastrointestinal side-effects will otherwise interfere with absorption of the drug. Hence, this procedure may be useful in cases where the degree of cervical ripeness or the presence of some spontaneous contractility indicates a high uterine sensitivity. So far there is only a limited experience with this approach [30], but the poor success rate with long induction–delivery intervals indicates that this approach is too ineffective to recommend it as routine management for a majority of cases.

On the basis of the literature and their own data, Karim et al. [1] have listed recommended dose schedules of prostaglandins given by different routes for the management of intrauterine foetal death. Our modification of these recommendations is presented in Table 4. In general our dose schedules correspond to those of Karim et al. [1], but correct some obvious mistakes such as extra-amniotic infusion of as much as 25 $\mu$g $PGE_2$/min. In addition we cannot recommend different dose schedules for use below and above 28 weeks of gestation, but prefer to start with the lower dosage and to increase it depending on the uterine response (Table 4).

*Prostaglandin analogues*

As discussed elsewhere (Embrey, chapter 13), there is a strong tendency to abandon systemic administration of natural prostaglandins in favour of either local administration or the use of analogues for termination of second

*Table 4.* Recommended dose schedules of natural prostaglandins given by different routes for the management of intrauterine foetal death (Modified after Karim et al. (1)).

| Route of administration[1] | Prostaglandin $E_2$ | Prostaglandin $F_{2\alpha}$ |
| --- | --- | --- |
| Intravenous infusion | 0.25–4 $\mu$g/min | 2.5–40 $\mu$g/min |
| Extra-amniotic infusion | 0.5–4 $\mu$g/min | 2.5–10$\mu$g/min[2] |
| Extra-amniotic doses | 25–200 $\mu$g every 2 h | 125–1000 $\mu$g every 2 h |
| Vaginal pessaries | 10–20 mg every 3–6 h | – |

[1] Intramuscular, oral and intra-amniotic routes are considered as not suitable (see text).
[2] Based on a very limited experience.

trimester pregnancies. As discussed above, local administration poses special problems in case of intrauterine foetal death. In addition, unlike other terminations, which can be referred to or grouped in centres with special expertise, the management of intrauterine death is often in the hands of gynaecologists with little or no experience of either prostaglandins or termination of pregnancy. Therefore, prostaglandin analogues that can overcome the relative need for local administration by longer half-lives and higher uterotonic specificity would be particularly suited to this situation. None of the prostaglandin analogues that have so far been tested can at present be described as the ideal compound for the future. As indicated elsewhere (Amy and Embrey, chapters 12 and 13) there is still considerable progress to be made with respect to both analogues and delivery systems. In the meantime some analogues already offer a suitable, though imperfect, solution for the problem at hand. In order to illustrate this point, Table 5 lists our personal experience, comparing extra-amniotic $PGF_{2\alpha}$ with systemic administration of a $PGF_{2\alpha}$ and a $PGE_2$ analogue according to original recommendations of the manufacturers, which we do no longer follow since reducing the dosage to half does not impair the results [24, 31]. In the Table it can be seen that 15(S),15-methyl-prostaglandin $F_{2\alpha}$ (15-me-$PGF_{2\alpha}$) is highly effective with the shortest induction–delivery intervals but at the expense of a high incidence of gastrointestinal side-effects. With 16-phenoxy-17,18,19,20-tetranor-prostaglandin $E_2$ methylsulphonylamide (sulprostone)gastrointestinal side-effects were less frequent, though more frequent than with extra-amniotic $PGF_{2\alpha}$. On the other hand, the induction-delivery interval became substantially longer and pyrexia was more frequent than in the other groups, which were comparable with respect to gestational age, parity and — in the case of 15-me-$PGF_{2\alpha}$ – duration of foetal death. In addition, there was a greater need for analgesia with intravenous sulprostone than with either one of the other approaches. It should be realized, however, that the doses of the analogues used in this and in many other studies (Table 6) are too high.

In a large multicentre trial [24] we found doses of 250 μg and 125 μg 15-me-PGF$_{2\alpha}$ administered every 2 h to be equally effective for terminating pregnancy after foetal death. There was no statistical difference in the incidence of side-effects either. This indicates that the dose of 250 μg which is commonly recommended for the termination of second trimester pregnancy may profitably be reduced to half and possibly even further when dealing with foetal death. The same appears to apply for intravenous sulprostone, for Gruber and Baumgarten [31] infused sulprostone at a rate of 0.25–2 μg/min in 10 patients reaching a mean induction–delivery interval of 8.8 h and a mean total dose of 845 μg as compared to our data (Table 5) which averaged at respectively 19.3 h and 1650 μg. Fawzy and Basioni [10] used an infusion rate of 100 μg/h and although their data are too poorly presented in order to judge

Table 5 Comparison of extra-amniotic PGF$_{2\alpha}$, intramuscular 15(S), 15-methyl-prostaglandin F$_{2\alpha}$ (15-me-PGF$_{2\alpha}$) and intravenous 16-phenoxy-17,18,19,20-tetranor-prostaglandin E$_2$ methylsulphonylamide (sulprostone) in the management of intrauterine foetal death

| Patients' data and criteria | Extra-amniotic PGF$_{2\alpha}$ (n = 15) | Intramuscular 15-me-PGF$_{2\alpha}$ (n = 15) | Intravenous sulprostone (n = 15) |
|---|---|---|---|
| Dose schedule | 0 5 mg initial dose, 0 25–1 0 mg every hour | 0 25 mg every 2 h | 1 5 mg/6h, eventually repeated after 24 h |
| No of nulliparous + parous patients | 5 + 10 | 4 + 11 | 6 + 9 |
| Gestational age in weeks median and (range) | 29 (18–39) | 29 (19–39) | 28 5 (19–38) |
| Duration of foetal death in days median and (range) | 7 (1–35) | 4 (1–28) | 3 (1–28) |
| Induction–delivery interval in hours median and (range) | 14 5 (7–36) | 6 8 (1 3–24 5) | 19 3 (6 2–3 1) |
| Total dose (in mg) required median and (range) | 8 (3–22 9) | 1 (0 25–3) | 1 5 (1 5–2 5) |
| No without retained products | 12 | 11 | 12 |
| Total loss of blood in ml median and (range) | 150 (20–870) | 50 (20–450) | 50 (20–510) |
| No with temperature ≥ 38° C | 0 | 0 | 4 |
| No with gastrointestinal side-effects | | | |
| No side-effects | 11 | 1 | 7 |
| Nausea only | 3 | 2 | 2 |
| Vomiting | 1 | 12 | 6 |
| Diarrhoea | 0 | 7 | 2 |

*Table 6* Termination of pregnancy in cases of intrauterine foetal death with intramuscular administration of prostaglandin analogues

| No of cases | No success fully treated | Gestation (weeks) | Dose | Induction delivery interval (h min) Mean | Range | Incidence (%) Vomiting | Diarr | Reference |
|---|---|---|---|---|---|---|---|---|
| | | | | | | | | |

<table>
<tr><td>No of cases</td><td>No success fully treated</td><td>Gestation (weeks)</td><td>Dose</td><td colspan="2">Induction delivery interval (h min)</td><td colspan="2">Incidence (%)</td><td>Reference</td></tr>
<tr><td></td><td></td><td></td><td></td><td>Mean</td><td>Range</td><td>Vomiting</td><td>Diarr</td><td></td></tr>
<tr><td colspan="9">2a,2b-dihomo-15(S),14-methyl-PGF<sub>2α</sub> methyl ester</td></tr>
<tr><td>24</td><td>23</td><td>15–28</td><td>500 μg every</td><td>12 04</td><td>1 55–29</td><td>13</td><td>0</td><td>Karim and</td></tr>
<tr><td>26</td><td>26</td><td>29–44</td><td>8h</td><td>11 04</td><td>2 50–32</td><td>12</td><td>0</td><td>Ratnam (32)</td></tr>
<tr><td colspan="9">15(S) 15-methyl-PGF<sub>2α</sub> (15-me-PGF<sub>2α</sub>)</td></tr>
<tr><td>52</td><td>52</td><td rowspan="2">14–40</td><td>125 μg every 2 h</td><td>–*</td><td>2 10–35 50</td><td>48</td><td>62</td><td>Wallenburg et al (24)</td></tr>
<tr><td>45</td><td>44</td><td>250 μg every 2 h</td><td>–*</td><td>0 25–20 20</td><td>56</td><td>56</td><td></td></tr>
<tr><td>58</td><td>58</td><td>12–27</td><td>250 μg every</td><td>7 50</td><td>1 00–21 30</td><td>40</td><td>35</td><td>De Gezelle</td></tr>
<tr><td>20</td><td>19</td><td>28–38</td><td>1–3 h</td><td>9 14</td><td>2 00–25 35</td><td>50</td><td>35</td><td>et al (33)</td></tr>
<tr><td colspan="9">16-phenoxy-17,18 19 20-tetranor-PGE<sub>2</sub>-methylsulphonylamide (sulprostone)</td></tr>
<tr><td>30</td><td>29</td><td>14–30</td><td>500 μg every</td><td>9 28</td><td>0 30–24 00</td><td>10</td><td>13</td><td>Karim et al</td></tr>
<tr><td>19</td><td>19</td><td>30–42</td><td>6 h</td><td>9 20</td><td>2 00–19 00</td><td>11</td><td>0</td><td>(34)</td></tr>
</table>

\* Mean values not given, median values equalled 13 4 and 7 3 h, respectively for nulliparous and parous women in the 125 μg group and 9 0 and 7 2 h in the 250 μg group

the results adequately, it would appear that they too obtained better results with lower doses than we did The firm conclusion that can be reached from the data that are now available is that for prostaglandin analogues too, dose–effect relationships will need to be established more carefully than has been the case so far, and separately from those applicable to other terminations in the second trimester With the lowering incidence of foetal death, future developments in this area will more than before depend on multicentre trials and a high level of collaboration among individual investigators

In the meantime intravenous infusion rates of sulprostone should probably not exceed 2 μg/min In our experience patients usually prefer intramuscular administration and this route of administration has so far been tested for three analogues The results of studies that have reported on at least 20 cases are summarised in Table 6 Our own experience is limited to 15-me-PGF$_{2α}$ and sulprostone From that experience, which is also limited, it is likely the doses of 125 μg 15-me-PGF$_{2α}$ every 2 to 3 h or 250 μg sulprostone every 4 to 6 h will be adequate in the majority of cases

*The influence of parity, gestational age and duration of foetal death*

It is generally acknowledged that the pregnant uterus is more responsive to prostaglandin stimulation than the nonpregnant one, and that the uterus requires a smaller total dose to initiate labour at term than at an earlier stage of pregnancy [35]. Similarly it is well known that multiparae require smaller doses than nulliparae for induction of labour [36], and it has been indicated above that the cause (Table 1) and duration of foetal death (Table 2) may influence the interval till delivery. This may well reflect a varying degree of uterine responsiveness. However, it is not yet clear to what extent these factors may influence the management of intrauterine foetal death.

In our multicentre trial using two dose schedules of 15-me-PGF$_{2\alpha}$ [24] we found that nulliparous women required a consistently higher dose and had longer induction–delivery intervals than parous women (Fig. 1). This is by no means a uniform finding, for Fawzy and Basioni [10] reported mean infusion–delivery times with sulprostone which were on the average lower for nulliparous than multiparous patients. Unfortunately, this study is so poorly reported, mixing patients with foetal death with cases of hydatidiform mole among other deficiencies, that it is not possible to analyse the results adequately. However, these authors reported mean intervals of 8.6 and 7.8 h in

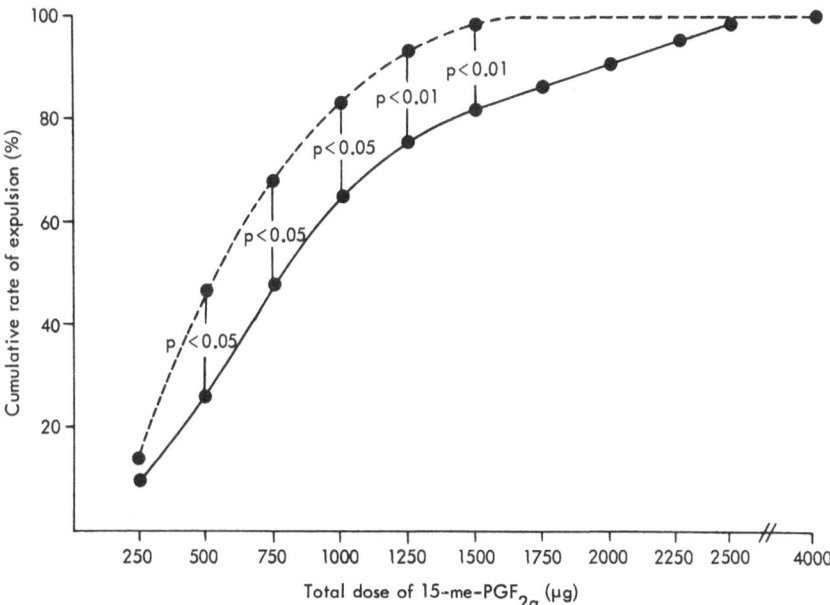

*Fig. 1.* Cumulative expulsion rates of the conceptus in relation to the total doses of 15-me-PGF$_{2\alpha}$ administered to 61 parous (– – –) and 35 nulliparous (———) women. 15-me-PGF$_{2\alpha}$ was administered in intramuscular doses of 125 $\mu$g or 250 $\mu$g every 2 h. Fisher and $\chi^2$ tests were used for statistical analysis. (From Wallenburg et al. (24).)

nulliparous women below and above 28 weeks respectively, as compared to 13.2 and 12.3 h in multiparous patients. Judging from the merit of the paper and the quality of the investigation, which resulted in a live-born foetal death, it is of course possible that the data were just interchanged. Nevertheless, to our knowledge no other studies have presently shown a statistically significant difference between nulliparous and parous patients in either doses required or induction–delivery intervals.

From many of the initial studies which used intravenous $PGE_2$ or $PGF_{2\alpha}$ one could draw the conclusion that at gestational ages above 28 weeks, pregnancy could be terminated with lower doses and/or shorter induction–delivery intervals than below 28 weeks [1]. As indicated above this led Karim et al. [1] to recommend different dose schedules for these two categories. The more recent studies based on both a larger number of cases and other approaches do not confirm the validity of a 28 weeks cut-off point as shown in Table 7. We have repeatedly found [12, 23, 24] that gestational age had no significant influence on induction–delivery intervals. Schulman et al. [9] reported the reverse in that they found that dosage requirements of vaginal

Table 7. Comparison of similar doses of prostaglandin for the management of so-called missed abortion (<28 weeks) and missed labour ($\geqslant$28 weeks). There is no evidence that induction–delivery intervals are shorter in cases of missed labour.

| Prostaglandin and dose used | Induction–delivery interval (h: min); mean and range | | References |
|---|---|---|---|
| | Missed abortion (n = 167) | Missed labour (n = 120) | |
| Extra-amniotic $PGF_{2\alpha}$ 0.5 mg initial dose; 0.25–1.10 mg/h | 14:56 (7:00–24:00) (n = 5) | 15:44 (7:20–36:00) (n = 10) | Luengo et al. (23) |
| 2a,2b-dihomo-15-me-$PGF_{2\alpha}$ methyl ester IM; 0.5 mg/8 h | 12:04 (1:55–29:00) (n = 23) | 11:04 (2:50–32:00) (n = 26) | Karim and Ratnam (32) |
| 15-me-$PGF_{2\alpha}$ IM; 0.1–0.25 mg/2–4 h | 4:30 (0:45–10:00) (n = 6) | 6:20 (4:00–20:00) (n = 7) | Ylikorkala et al. (37) |
| 15-me-$PGF_{2\alpha}$ IM; 0.25 mg/1–3 h | 7:50 (1:00–21:30) (n = 58) | 9:14 (2:00–25:35) (n = 19) | De Gezelle et al. (33) |
| 15-me-$PGF_{2\alpha}$ IM; 0.25 mg/2 h | 8:36 (0:30–19:30) (n = 17) | 8:03 (0:25–20:20) (n = 27) | Wallenburg et al. (24)[1] |
| Vaginal $PGE_2$; 20 mg/2–5 h | 8:19 (1:15–15:30) (n = 29) | 11:01 (4:45–24:30) (n = 12) | Thiery et al. (38) |
| Sulprostone IM; 0.5 mg/6 h | 9:28 (0:30–24:00) (n = 29) | 9:20 (2:00–19:00) (n = 19) | Karim et al. (34) |

[1] Mean intervals and gestational ages were recalculated from the original data.

$PGE_2$ decreased progressively with gestational age. However, mean doses in the gestational groups between 20 and 37 weeks were similar ranging from 40 to 34 mg, and the difference is created by cases below 20 weeks, all of which resulted from failed induced abortions. This is hardly representative for the usual cases of foetal death and indicates how deeply the habit of mixing apples with oranges is imbedded in current clinical investigations.

When speculating on future developments, we expect that earlier gestations may well require either higher doses or longer induction–delivery intervals, although our results do not substantiate it. This would be consistent with an increasing uterine sensitivity during pregnancy, the relation between oxytocin sensitivity and the required doses of prostaglandins after foetal death [9], and shorter intervals between foetal death and delivery with advancing gestational age (Table 2). Nevertheless, such a difference will have to be clearly demonstrated in order to justify differential dose schedules. From the evidence available (Table 7) there is certainly no reason to presume that the 28 weeks threshold will become a valuable cut-off point.

Another question that needs to be considered is whether the cause and/or duration of foetal death may influence induction-delivery intervals. Van Iddelkinge and Gordon [39] found that doses of intravenous $PGE_2$ required for the management of intrauterine death were significantly lower in cases of placental insufficiency than in cases of rhesus isoimmunization. This would be consistent with older data on the interval between foetal death and expulsion shown in Table 1, but to our knowledge these observations have not been confirmed. In a large multicentre trial, Southern et al. [29] found the total doses of vaginal $PGE_2$ and induction–delivery intervals to be longer when the foetus had been retained in utero for 3 weeks or more. El-Damarawy et al. [40] reached similar conclusions with vaginal $PGE_2$ and suggested that there is a positive correlation between the duration of foetal death and induction–delivery intervals. In our studies [12, 23, 24] we have been unable to confirm such a relationship, though this may be due to the fact that cases with prolonged retention of a dead foetus are rare in our population. This in turn is due to characteristics of antenatal care in our community and to our active approach to the management of foetal death. From the combined evidence, however, it is clear that induction of labour, when deemed necessary, will not be facilitated by a preceding episode of expectant management, although it is possible of course that in a number of cases labour will have ensued spontaneously in the meantime.

CONCLUSIONS

Attitudes towards the management of intrauterine death have certainly changed over the past few decades. During the last decade in particular, there has been a strong tendency to abandon the time-honoured therapy of procrastination in favour of a more active approach. The main resons for this change are a greater insistence on the patient's emotional needs and wishes and the availability of more adequate means to terminate such pregnancies. Advances in perinatal medicine have drastically lowered the incidence of foetal death late in pregnancy and have brought about other changes that may be equally important. A greater proportion of intrauterine deaths now occur earlier in pregnancy: more than 50% before 28 and more than 90% before 37 weeks. As well as occurring earlier, these deaths are suspected earlier and diagnosed earlier, at a time when the end of pregnancy appears to be a long way off.

While there can be no doubt that prostaglandins given by various routes are highly effective for the termination of such pregnancies, the choice of the compound and the route of administration will finally depend on what compound is available in what country. There are only a few countries, such as the United Kingdom, where the choice between $PGE_2$ and $PGF_{2\alpha}$ is not dictated by their availability. For the next decade or so this will continue to apply to the more potent prostaglandin analogues. However, the experience so far is promising. Some analogues already provide an effective approach with a minimum of risks, although the frequency of gastrointestinal side-effects remains a matter of major concern. Much of this can be reduced by adequate premedication, but premedication remains a rather poor substitute for better analogues and delivery systems by which its use may be avoided altogether.

In the meantime the somatic nuisances of relatively short duration should be weighed against the possibly prolonged psychosocial impact of procrastination. In order to do so, it is essential to present the patient with the alternative choices. It is equally important to have an adequate follow-up that includes both medical aspects and the patient's satisfaction. Since our department adopted that policy, proponents of procrastination have become miraculously extinct, which does not imply that we have been able to make the termination of such pregnancies an easy and agreeable routine procedure.

REFERENCES

1　Karim SMM, Ng SC and Ratnam SS Termination of abnormal intrauterine pregnancy with prostaglandins In *Practical Applications of Prostaglandins and their Synthesis Inhibitors*, Karim SMM (ed), pp 319–374 MTP, Lancaster, 1979
2　FIGO News Lists of gynecologic and obstetrical terms and difinitions *Int J Gynaecol Obstet* 14 570–576, 1976

153

3  WHO  Recommended definitions, terminology and format for statistical tables related to perinatal period and use of a new certificate for cause of perinatal deaths  *Acta Obstet Gynecol Scand* 56  247–253, 1977

4  Butler NR and Alberman ED (eds)  *Perinatal Problems*  Livingstone, Edinburgh-London, 1969

5  Keirse MJNC  Epidemiology of pre-term labour  In  *Human Parturition  New Concepts and Developments*, Keirse MJNC, Anderson ABM and Bennebroek Gravenhorst J (eds), pp 219–234  Leiden University Press, The Hague, 1979

6  Grandin DJ and Hall RE  Fetal death before the onset of labor  An analysis of 407 cases  *Am J Obstet Gynecol* 79  237–243, 1960

7  Tricomi V and Kohl SG  Fetal death in utero  *Am J Obstet Gynecol* 74  1092–1097, 1957

8  Csapo AI  The 'see-saw' theory of parturition  In  *The Fetus and Birth*, pp  159–195  Ciba Foundation Symposium no  47, Elsevier, Amsterdam, 1977

9  Schulman H, Saldana L, Lin CC and Randolph G  Mechanism of failed labor after fetal death and its treatment with prostaglandin $E_2$  *Am J Obstet Gynecol* 133  742–752, 1979

10  Fawzy A and Basiony BA  The use of sulprostone in the management of death in utero and molar pregnancy  *Singapore J Obstet Gynaecol* 10  39–42, 1979

11  Pritchard JA  Fetal death in utero  *Obstet Gynecol* 14  573–580, 1959

12  Keirse MJNC and Bennebroek Gravenhorst J  Het inleiden van de baring bij intrauteriene vruchtdood  *Ned Tijdschr Geneesk* 123  1195–1199, 1975

13  Donald I  *Practical Obstetric Problems*  Lloyd-Luke, London, 1969

14  Martin RH and Menzies DN  Oestrogen therapy in missed abortion and labour  *J Obstet Gynaecol Br Emp* 62  256–258, 1955

15  Courtney LD, Boxall RR and Child P  Permeability of membranes of dead fetus  *Br med J* 1  492–493, 1971

16  Loudon JDO  The use of high concentration oxytocin intravenous drips in the management of missed abortion  *J Obstet Gynaecol Br Emp* 66  277–281, 1959

17  Liggins GC  The treatment of missed abortion by high dosage Syntocinon intravenous infusion  *J Obstet Gynaecol Br Commonw* 69  227–281, 1962

18  Ursell W  Induction of labour following fetal death  *J Obstet Gynaecol Br Commonw* 79  260–264, 1972

19  Karim SSM  The use of prostaglandin $E_2$ in the management of missed abortion, missed labour and hydatidiform mole  *Br Med J* 3  196–197, 1970

20  Moe N  The intravenous infusion of prostaglandin $F_{2\alpha}$ in the management of intrauterine death of the fetus  *Acta Obstet Gynecol Scand* 55  113–114, 1976

21  Briel RC, Kunz S and Kidess E  Beeinflussung der Hamostase bei Missed Abortion durch Prostaglandin $F_{2\alpha}$  *Geburtshilfe Frauenheilkd* 38  862–867, 1978

22  Keirse MJNC, Bennebroek Gravenhorst J, Boekhout-Mussert MJ, Dubbeldam J and Veltkamp JJ  Coagulation changes during management of fetal death with 15(S)-15-methyl-prostaglandin $F_{2\alpha}$  *Eur J Obstet Gynecol Reprod Biol* 11  43–48, 1980

23  Luengo J, Keirse MJNC and Bennebroek Gravenhorst J  Extra amniotic prostaglandin $F_{2\alpha}$ for intra-uterine death and fetal abnormality  *Eur J Obstet Gynecol Reprod Biol* 7  325–329, 1977

24  Wallenburg HCS, Keirse MJNC, Freie HMP and Blacquiere JF  Intramuscular administration of 15(S)-15-methyl-prostaglandin $F_{2\alpha}$ for induction of labour in patients with fetal death  *Br J Obstet Gynaecol* 87  203–209, 1980

25  Keirse MJNC, Williamson JG and Turnbull AC  Metabolism of prostaglandin $F_{2\alpha}$ within the human uterus in early pregnancy  *Br J Obstet Gynaecol* 82  142–145, 1975

26  Keirse MJNC and Turnbull AC  Metabolism of prostaglandins within the pregnant uterus  *Br J Obstet Gynaecol* 82  887–893, 1975

27  Keirse MJNC  15(S),15-methyl-prostaglandin $F_{2\alpha}$ in the management of intrauterine fetal death  In  *Prostaglandins and Thromboxanes*, Forster W (ed), pp  463–466  Gustav Fischer, Jena, 1981

28  Karim SMM  Prostaglandins and human reproduction  physiological roles and clinical use of prostaglandins in relation to human reproduction  In  *The Prostaglandins  Progress in Research*, Karim SMM (ed), pp  71–164  MTP, Lancaster, 1972

154

29  Southern EM, Gutknecht GD, Mohberg NR and Edelman DA  Vaginal prostaglandin $E_2$ in the management of fetal intrauterine dealth  *Br J Obstet Gynaecol* 85  437–441, 1978

30  Kho FHG and de Bruin AJJ  The use of oral prostaglandin $E_2$ in the management of intrauterine fetal death  *Prostaglandins* 18  663–672, 1979

31  Gruber WS and Baumgarten K  Intravenous prostaglandin $E_2$ and 16-phenoxy prostaglandin $E_2$ methyl sulfonamide for induction of fetal death in utero  *Am J Obstet Gynecol* 137  8–14, 1980

32  Karim SMM and Ratnam SS  Termination of abnormal intrauterine pregnancies with intramuscular administration of dihomo 15 methyl prostaglandin $F_{2\alpha}$  *Br J Obstet Gynaecol* 83  885–889, 1976

33  De Gezelle H, Thiery M, Parewijck W and Decoster JM  Prostaglandin $F_{2\alpha}$ for interrupting pregnancy, managing intrauterine death and molar pregnancy and induced labor  *Int J Gynaecol Obstet* 17  362–367, 1980

34  Karim SMM, Lim AL, Prasad RNV, Yeo KC, Ng SC, Salmon YM, Choo HT and Ratnam SS  Termination of abnormal intrauterine pregnancy with intramuscular administration of sulprostone  *Singapore J Obstet Gynaecol* 10  33–37, 1979

35  Embrey MP  *Prostaglandins in reproduction*  Churchill, London, 1975

36  Keirse MJNC, Sokolewicz JJ, Frankena A and Jaszmann L  Comparison of oral prostaglandin $E_2$ and intravenous oxytocin for induction of labor in hypertensive pregnancy  *Eur J Obstet Gynecol Reprod Biol* 10  231–237, 1980

37  Ylikorkala O, Kirkinen P and Jarvinen PA  Intramuscular administration of 15-methyl-prostaglandin $F_{2\alpha}$ for induction of labour in patients with intrauterine fetal death or an anencephalic fetus  *Br J Obstet Gynaecol* 83  502–504, 1976

38  Thiery M, Amy JJ and Decoster JM  Vaginal prostaglandin $E_2$ for interruption of pregnancy and management of intrauterine death  *Z Geburtshilfe Perinatol* 183  218–222, 1979

39  Van Iddelkinge B and Gordon H  cited by Karim et al (1)

40  El-Damarawy H, El-Sahwi S and Toppozada M  Management of missed abortion and fetal death in utero  *Prostaglandins* 14  583–590, 1977

# 15. COMPLICATIONS OF SECOND TRIMESTER ABORTION

Gary S. Berger, and Louis G. Keith

Abortion is one of the most prevalent means of fertility control in use throughout the world. In the United States alone, over one million abortions were performed in 1977 [1]. It is estimated that more than 30 million abortions are performed annually on a world-wide basis [2]. In some countries, abortions are obtained legally; in many parts of the world, however, abortion remains a criminal or clandestine operation. Only in the last decade have data generally become available from Western Europe and the United States regarding the incidence and types of complications associated with abortion performed under legal sanction. Data regarding the complications of illegal abortions remain fragmentary and inferential. For example, it is known that deaths from complications are frequent in countries where abortion is illegal, but their numbers only reflect one aspect of the problem i.e., that which is obvious and cannot be hidden. The true numbers of illegal procedures and the extent of the associated morbidity remain unknown.

Even in countries where abortion is a legal operation, complications occur in the hands of the best trained and most experienced physicians. Because of the number of women undergoing abortion, these complications may represent a substantial public health problem. In 1975, in the United States alone an estimated 77 000 women had abortion related complications and 29 deaths resulted from abortion. The direct cost of treating these complications was estimated to be over $ 19 million [3]. In sharp contrast, among 700 000 abortions performed in the Netherlands over the last several years only 1 death occurred, and the general level of morbidity was lower than in the United States during a comparable time (Ketting, personal communication, 1980).

The three factors which are directly related to the morbidity of abortion are: 1) gestational age, 2) abortion technique, and 3) the experience and training of the physician. The most important indirect factor which reflects abortion morbidity is the presence or absence of an ongoing internal monitoring system to detect problems as they arise. These factors, as they relate to abortion morbidity and specific complications associated with second trimester abortion procedures, will be discussed in this chapter.

*M.J.N.C. Keirse et al. (eds.), Second Trimester Pregnancy Termination. All rights reserved*
*Copyright © 1982 Martinus Nijhoff Publishers, The Hague/Boston/London.*

156

Abortion morbidity (both the rates of major and minor complications) clearly increases with increasing gestational age [3–5]. The rates of major complications rapidly increase from about 0.3 per 100 abortions at 7–8 menstrual weeks gestation to 2.26 per 100 abortions at 21–24 menstrual weeks gestation. This increase must be viewed as a continuum, since there is no specific time, e.g. between the first and second trimester, when the rate increases more rapidly than before. This concept is substantiated in a number of studies and is clinically significant because it is clear that *any* delay in obtaining an abortion places the patient at an increased risk.

Although the use of menstrual extraction or very early suction curettage before pregnancy can be diagnosed reliably may result in some nonpregnant women undergoing a uterine evacuation procedure, the morbidity of such procedures is minimal [6]. Continuing efforts must be made to educate women as well as the medical profession and abortion referral services about the increased risks of abortion associated with advancing gestational age.

## TECHNIQUE OF ABORTION

Since the choice of abortion technique is related to gestational age, for many years clinicians chose to restrict the use of uterine evacuation procedures using suction and/or sharp curettage to gestations of 12–14 menstrual (10–12) conceptional) weeks or less. Beyond 12–14 weeks gestation, many clinicians have chosen to delay abortion procedures until after 16 or more menstrual weeks gestation and then treat the patient by the intra-amniotic instillation of an abortifacient, usually hypertonic saline. A number of more recent reports, however, from America and Europe have demonstrated that uterine evacuation procedures can safely be used for terminating pregnancies from 16 to 22 menstrual weeks gestation [7, 8]. The question of comparative safety of midtrimester procedures has been considered by Grimes and Cates (chapter 7). Brenner and Edelman [9] also are of the opinion that a uterine evacuation procedure (D&E — dilation and evacuation) at 12–15 weeks gestation is safer than waiting until after 15 weeks and using an instillation procedure. It is this 'grey zone' between 13 and 17 menstrual weeks gestation which has presented considerable problems to clinicians in the past. Many authorities believe that adherence to a policy of 'no treatment' during this time artificially causes a delay for many women from late first trimester into the second trimester, thus exposing them to additional risk. Continuing concern regarding comparative safety of different procedures at various gestational ages is shared by a great number of international authorities. At late gestational ages

157

there are numerous individual advocates of a variety of specific nonsurgical evacuation procedures including intra-amniotic administration of hypertonic saline, urea, or natural prostaglandins or their analogues and the intra-muscular or extra-amniotic administration of prostaglandin analogues.

PHYSICIAN TRAINING AND EXPERIENCE

As with any surgical procedure, the skill and experience of the physician, the level of prior training, and certain innate abilities all affect the outcome of the procedure, including the management of complications. To date, the medical community generally has not adequately evaluated physician-related variables in terms of the associated complication rates of the abortion proce-dures. The wide range of complication rates reported for similar abortion procedures at different hospitals and clinics may be more a function of the individual physician concerned than of differences in abortion techniques or characteristics of women undergoing abortion. Bozorgi's [10] analysis of more than 10 000 procedures and Burnhill's [11] reports from the Preterm Institute stand out in that they assessed complications by specific physicians. Only rarely does the published literature address the problem of physician competence and internal methods of quality control in abortion clinics [8, 12]. For the sake of all concerned, those physicians who experience extremely high rates of complications should either acquire additional training and improved skills or refrain from performing abortions.

SECOND TRIMESTER ABORTION COMPLICATIONS

While the incidence of complications is related to gestational age, abortion technique and training and experience of the physician, the occurrence of specific types of complications is primarily related to the abortion technique itself. Table 1 lists some of the major complications of second trimester abortion procedures.

*Uterine Perforation/Injury*

Although the risk of uterine perforation rapidly increases with gestational age, the magnitude of this increased risk is small – from less than 0.2% for first trimester procedures to about 0.3–0.4% for second trimester procedures.

Not all perforations, either suspected or confirmed, require treatment. Perforations caused by blunt instruments, e.g., sound or dilator, can be 'treated' more frequently by observing the patient than is the case with

*Table 1.* Major abortion complications.

---

*Immediate complications*
Uterine perforation/injury
Cervical injury
Hemorrhage
Anesthesia
Coagulation defects
Hypernatremia
Water intoxication
Failed abortion
Incomplete abortion

*Delayed complications*
Retained products of conception
Infection
Rh Sensitization
Reproductive failure

---

perforations caused by sharp or suction curettes. Except in emergencies where severe loss of blood is obvious, laparoscopy is recommended for evaluation of the severity of the uterine perforation. Its use may eliminate the need for exploratory laparotomy or prolonged hospitalization for observation. Damage from perforation may be life threatening if a branch of the uterine artery is lacerated at the time of perforation. The anatomic variations of the branches of the uterine artery are often considerable. Since these branches are directly 'on line' with the aorta via their source, the internal iliac artery, any loss of blood from a laceration of even a minor branch of the uterine artery may be severe. Therapy of each case must be individualized. In some instances, the prompt use of bilateral hypogastric artery ligation will avoid the necessity of a hysterectomy [13].

Uterine injuries occurring in conjunction with instillation procedures are fortunately a rare event. Cases of cervical or uterine rupture have been reported; the former are associated with use of prostaglandins and the latter often result from overstimulation of the uterus with oxytocic agents.

*Cervical injury*

The risk of cervical injury is somewhat higher for second than for first trimester surgical evacuation procedures. The average rate for second trimester procedures is about 1.1% (range 0.0–7.1%) [14]. In reports on large series of first trimester abortions, on the other hand, the reported rates are usually less than 1% [10].

Cervical injuries usually occur during dilatation of the cervix and frequently result from traction on the tenaculum. Lacerations from tenacula may be treated by cervical suturing or by firm packing against the cervix to control bleeding. Cervical perforations with the sound, dilator or curette are rare but can reach a branch of the uterine artery.

Potentially more serious cervical injuries occur in conjunction with non-surgical abortion procedures. These range from simple cervical lacerations or tears to cervicovaginal fistulae. Many result from the rapid expulsion of the products of conception through an inadequately dilated cervix. Rates of cervical injury of about 0.5% have been reported in association with saline and prostaglandin $F_{2\alpha}$-induced abortions ]15].

For both surgical and nonsurgical abortion procedures, the risk of cervical injury may be reduced by predilating the cervix with laminaria or pharmacological agents (e.g. prostaglandins) before initiation of the abortion procedure.

*Hemorrhage*

Hemorrhage is a complication which can occur with any of the presently available second trimester abortion procedures. One problem in evaluating hemorrhage rates for different abortion procedures reported by different investigators is that inconsistent definitions of hemorrhage are used and the methods of estimating the amount of blood lost are usually totally inadequate. A more objective measure of the severity of the hemorrhage is the need for blood transfusions, but use of this as the sole criteria does not address the continuing problem of physicians performing abortions, i.e. accurately estimating the blood loss in individual cases. Rates of hemorrhage requiring transfusion appear to be lower for D&E procedures (0.2%) than for either intra-amniotic saline (1.0%) or prostaglandin $F_{2\alpha}$ (1.5%) [3].

Excessive hemorrhage usually is associated with injury to one of the major uterine blood vessels or with placental separation, retained placenta or uterine atony. Berger and Kerenyi [16] found that the incidence of hemorrhage for saline-induced abortions increased with increasing duration of placental retention following abortion of the fetus. To reduce abortion morbidity these investigators recommended either surgical or manual removal of the placenta if it did not deliver spontaneously within two hours of the fetus. A drastic reduction in late complication rates may be obtained if manual curage and ring forceps evacuation of the uterus is routinely performed after instillation procedures to remove retained tissues.

*Anesthesia*

For first trimester suction curettage abortions, the overall rates of major complications are similar for abortions performed under local (paracervical) or general anesthesia [17]. Rates of specific complications, however, differ for the two anesthetic procedures. General anesthesia is associated with higher rates of hemorrhage, uterine perforation and cervical injury. Paracervical block anesthesia is associated with higher rates of post-operative fever and convulsions.

Whether similar findings will be applicable to second trimester D&E procedures remains to be demonstrated. At present, there is no consensus regarding which method is preferable. American [10] and Dutch [8] physicians who routinely perform D&E presently favor local anesthesia. Some physicians from the United Kingdom, on the other hand, prefer general anesthesia (Finks, personal communication, 1980).

Complications from paracervical block anesthesia are for the most part either preventable or easily treated. Paracervical anesthesia may have an additional benefit of reducing the likelihood of vasovagal reactions, especially if adrenaline is added to the anesthetic solution [8]. Specific techniques for placing the anesthetic agent into the cervix vary widely.

*Coagulation Defects*

Most women aborted with intra-amniotic saline demonstrate some coagulation defects [18]. For all but a few women, however, these coagulation defects are not clinically obvious and can only be determined through laboratory evaluations. Degradation products of fibrin and fibrinogen rise after saline instillation. Subsequently, there is a decrease in the platelet count, fibrinogen and Factor VIII levels. Changes in the coagulation system also occur after the administration of intra-amniotic urea [19]. Following the administration of prostaglandin $F_{2\alpha}$ an increase in platelets, fibrinogen and Factors V and VIII have been reported as well [20].

Although not generally recognized, disseminated intravascular coagulation has also been reported to occur following D&E procedures [21]. Available data presently suggest that this complication is less likely to occur after D&E than after saline- or urea-induced abortion.

*Hypernatremia*

Hypernatremia is a complication specific to saline abortion. Probably, intravascular injection is responsible for clinically significant hypernatremia. The incidence of this complication is less than 0.01 per 100 saline abortions and no deaths from abortion-related hypernatremia have been reported in the United States since 1972 [3].

*Water Intoxication*

Water intoxication is most often associated with high doses of oxytocin and the administration of large amounts of electrolyte-free solutions. This complication is entirely avoidable. If oxytocin is to be used to augment medically induced abortions, it should be administered in Ringer's solution or normal saline and the patient's fluid intake and output should be monitored closely.

*Failed Abortions*

Up to 2% of the women who have saline-, urea- or prostaglandin-induced abortions fail to abort the fetus. For these women, a repeat procedure or a different procedure is required. Even for abortions performed by D&E there is a small failure rate. Sometimes the physician is unable to introduce a suitably sized curet through the cervical canal or completely evacuate the products of conception because of uterine and/or cervical abnormalities. In such instances, it is advisable to stop and call for consultation. In the case of the undilated cervix, the risk of proceeding is either a major laceration or the creation of a false passage. In the case of incomplete evacuation, reevacuation under more favorable circumstances is in order — i.e. better anesthesia, special instruments, assistance of a more skilled colleague.

*Incomplete Abortion*

A frequent complication of all nonsurgical methods of abortion is failure to expel all products of conception following expulsion of the fetus. As a consequence, the placenta must often be removed by manual evacuation or by curettage [22]. It is not necessary to perform the curage or curettage under general anesthesia; the complications of such a procedure should be minimal since the cervix is already dilated and the placenta can usually be removed easily. Bieniarz (personal communication, 1980) has used a combination of curage and Ring forceps in his last several hundred cases with the patient at the end of the bed. His results have been excellent. Stubblefield (personal communication, 1980) has observed that these secondary evacuation procedures can be performed by junior staff under local sedation in a simple treatment room rather than in the operating room.

Rates of incomplete abortion are higher for saline than intra-amniotic prostaglandin $F_{2\alpha}$. Rates for saline range from 10 to 63% and for prostaglandin from 9 to 53% in individual investigations [23]. Berger and Kerenyi [16] found that complications (hemorrhage and/or infection) of saline-induced abortions increased with increasing duration of placental retention following expulsion of the fetus — from 2.5% if the placenta was expelled with the fetus to 8.2% if the placenta was retained for four or more hours.

*Retained Products of Conception*

After the abortion has been completed, there is still the possibility that some products of conception are retained in the uterus. The proportion of women initially aborted with a surgical procedure and undergoing a repeat curettage, increases with increasing gestational age until about 3% for second trimester procedures [4]. Most studies in the literature under-report rates of repeat curettage and other complications which occur after hospital/clinic discharge. Accurate reporting requires that women be followed up after their discharge from the hospital/clinic. Treatment is repeat curettage. Many physicians also administer therapeutic doses of antibiotics at the time of repeat curettage whether or not infection is clinically evident.

*Infection*

The determination of an abortion-related infection on the basis of elevated temperature alone is probably unsatisfactory, since many patients become febrile following the abortion with no other symptomatology. In most cases these fevers resolve spontaneously. Among 17 000 second trimester D&E procedures, the overall infection rate was 1.0% (range 0–3.8%) [14]. On the other hand, rates of pelvic infection following the intra-amniotic instillation of saline, prostaglandin $F_{2\alpha}$ or urea appear to be higher than for D&E procedures [15, 19]. These increased rates, in part, may reflect a reporting bias. Most D&E are performed as outpatient procedures and patients are discharged soon after completion of the procedures. In contrast, instillation abortions generally are performed as inpatient procedures and the patients are observed for longer periods of time. This bias is not corrected by follow-up of the patients, since the follow-up rate is usually low regardless of the type of abortion procedure.

*Rh Sensitization*

Rh sensitization after abortion is a preventable complication (Bennebroek Gravenhorst, chapter 16). The risk of sensitization increases with increasing gestational age, and *all* Rh negative, unsensitized women should be administered Rh immune globulin as prophylaxis after any abortion procedure. The magnitude of the risk of sensitization has not been adequately defined for second trimester procedures, although significant feto-maternal hemorrhages occur in more than 10% of late D&E abortions. The required dose of Rh immune globulin probably depends on the length of gestation; but to date a gestational age dependent dose schedule has not been worked out [24]. After second trimester procedures, it is probably best to give a dose equivalent to that of term delivery, unless it can be demonstrated that more is needed because of a massive feto-maternal hemorrhage. In the United States, this normal dose would be 300 $\mu$g. The most commonly used American product is Rhogam (Ortho Diagnostics, Raritan, NJ.).

*Reproductive Failure*

Questions regarding the effects of abortion on subsequent reproduction have not been adequately answered (Rowland Hogue, chapter 19). The relationships between various techniques of abortion, both surgical and nonsurgical, and subsequent spontaneous abortion, low birth weight, preterm birth, and cervical incompetence need to be evaluated further. The results of the presently available research on the subsequent effects of abortion — either by suction or by sharp curettage — generally indicate either a slightly greater or equal risk of spontaneous abortion, low birth weight or prematurity [25, 26]. Further work remains to be done to evaluate the late effects of nonsurgical methods of abortion and the incidence of cervical incompetence more completely.

MONITORING

Performance monitoring should be an integral part of the services of any clinic providing abortion services. The principal medical purpose of performance monitoring is to evaluate the quality of services provided to the patient. In some clinics, the monitoring task may be accomplished through the review of individual patient record forms. In larger-volume clinics, however, this type of monitoring becomes excessively time consuming and expensive and generally is not feasible. Under these circumstances, performance can best be monitored through the use of automated information retrieval systems.

A computerized data retrieval system using standardized data collection instruments can effectively provide the medical staff with information for evaluating all aspects of the abortion process. Although the monitoring of data in and of itself does not improve the quality of the abortion services, it can help upgrade patient services by providing information about specific areas. Suggested aspects of the total abortion procedure that should be monitored and evaluated include:

1. Preoperative patient counseling. Has the patient been informed as to what to expect during the abortion as well as during the postoperative course? Has she selected a method of contraception?

2. Laboratory tests. Have a pregnancy test, Papanicolaou smear, gonor-

rhea culture and blood typing been performed and the results documented for all patients?

3. Initiation of contraception. Which one has been selected? Any contraceptive method or sterilization may be safely initiated after an abortion (see Keith and Berger, chapter 17).

4. If the patient cannot be aborted at the clinic, have arrangements been made by the clinic for the patient to obtain the abortion elsewhere? The outcome for these patients should be known to the clinic personnel.

5. If the patient had an abnormal Papanicolaou smear or a positive gonorrhea culture or if any pathology was diagnosed at the clinic, was appropriate care given in the clinic or was the patient referred to another facility for treatment? Such patients should be followed to determine if the referral was completed. Since the results of Pap smears and gonorrhea cultures are not available until after the patient is discharged from the clinic, the clinic must be able to contact all patients with positive reports. In order to avoid the possibility of acute pelvic inflammatory disease, the patient whose gonorrhea culture is positive should be contacted and treated immediately upon receipt of the culture report. Except under the most unusual circumstances, this should be within 36–48 h after the culture was obtained. Patients should clearly understand the possible need for such follow-up and make mutually agreeable arrangements with clinic personnel for future contact, if required.

6. Review the morbidity and mortality and the number of patients requiring hospitalization or repeat abortion.

In general, abortion clinics have underutilized data management and information retrieval systems for the monitoring and evaluation of medical care. The technology for such systems has been available for many years, and the cost of implementing a clinical data management system are within the grasp of most clinics. The objectives of such an information system would be to:

1. Provide timely data on the activities and services provided.
2. Monitor the quality of medical care to ensure uniformity of standards.
3. Provide a socio-economic, demographic and reproductive profile of the clients.
4. Satisfy local, state and federal reporting requirements.

The system characteristics should include:

1. Accuracy – the data should be complete and should be free of errors.
2. Timeliness – the data should be up to date.
3. Effectiveness — the amount and type of data collected should be commensurate with the amount and type of information needed.
4. Flexibility — changes in the type and amount of data collected as well as the contents and frequency of reports should be relatively simple and easy to make.

5. Ease of data collection — the form of data acquisition should not impose undue hardship on the clinic staff.
6. Understandability — the format and contents of reports should be matched to the information needs and backgrounds of their intended audiences.

The minimum information that should be collected on each patient includes:
1. A socio-economic description.
2. Prior reproductive history.
3. Any history of medical or surgical abnormalities.
4. Any known allergies to medication.
5. A description of all services provided.
6. Results of laboratory tests such as GC, VDRL, Pap and Rh type.
7. Follow-up and documentation of treatment for abnormal tests.
8. Details of any immediate complications including the reasons for the complication, treatment rendered and outcome of treatment.
9. Details of any delayed complications including the reasons for the complication, treatment rendered and outcome of treatment.
10. Details of any hospitalization required.
11. The percentage of patients followed up and the relative characteristics of those with and without follow-up.

SUMMARY

Notwithstanding the experience and skill of the physicians performing the abortions, second trimester procedures, compared to first trimester abortions, still have an increased risk of significant morbidity, regardless of the abortion technique used. While the debate will continue as to what is the safest method of abortion, there is little doubt that the earlier it is performed the safer it is.

Given the limitations of today's knowledge and technology, the morbidity of abortion may be reduced if physicians pay careful attention to abortion technique and do not attempt to perform procedures for which they have not received the appropriate training. It is unfortunate that many university teaching services throughout the United States and Europe provide only minimal experience in abortion techniques to their young staff members. The system of preceptorship in special clinics which exists in Holland could well serve as a model for other countries.

166

ACKNOWLEDGEMENTS

Support for the preparation of this article was received from the Center for the Advancement of Reproductive Health, Chapel Hill, N C , and the Charles A Fields Medical Foundation, Ltd , Chicago, IL

REFERENCES

1 Center for Disease Control, United States Department of Health, Education and Welfare, Washington, DC *Abortion Surveillance 1977* HEW Publications, Atlanta, 6A, 1979
2 Tietze C and Lewit S Legal abortion *Sci Am* 236 21, 1977
3 Grimes DA and Cates W Complications from legally induced abortion a review *Obstet Gynecol Surv* 34 177, 1979
4 Edelman DA, Brenner WE and Berger, GS The effectiveness and complications of abortion by dilation and vacuum aspiration versus dilatation and rigid metal curettage *Am J Obstet Gynecol* 119 473, 1974
5 Stewart GK and Goldstein P Medical and surgical complications of therapeutic abortions *Obstet Gynecol* 40 539, 1972
6 Edelman DA and Berger GS Menstrual regulation *Techniques for Abortion and Sterilization*, Hodgson J (ed), Academic Press, in press
7 Hodari AA, Peralta J, Quiroga PJ and Gerbi ER Dilation and curettage for second trimester abortions *Am J Obstet Gynecol* 127 850, 1977
8 Van Lith DAF, Beekhuizen W and Van Schie KJ Complications of aspirotomy (AT) a modified dilatation and curettage procedure for terminating early second trimester pregnancies In *Pregnancy Termination*, Zatuchni GI, Sciarra JJ and Speidel JJ (eds), pp 193–205 Harper & Row, Hagerstown, MD, 1979
9 Brenner WE and Edelman DA Dilatation and evacuation at 13 to 15 weeks gestation versus intraamniotic saline after 15 weeks gestation *Contraception* 10 71, 1974
10 Bozorgi N Termination of pregnancy in a private outpatient clinic *Am J Obstet Gynecol* 127 763, 1977
11 Burnhill M *Physician Manual Standard Medical Procedures* Preterm Institute Newton MA, 1975
12 Keith L, Berger GS and Edelman DA Monitoring care in abortion clinics *J Reprod Med* 21 163–168, 1978
13 Keith L and Berger GS Surgical management of intractable pelvic hemorrhage In *Gynecology and Obstetrics*, II, 38, Sciarra JJ (ed) Harper & Row, Hagerstown MD 1977
14 Cates W, Schulz KF, Gold J and Tyler CW Complications of surgical evacuation procedures for abortions after 12 weeks gestation In *Pregnancy termination*, pp 206–217 Zatuchni GI, Sciarra JJ and Speidel JJ (eds), Harper & Row, Hagerstown, MD, 1979
15 Grimes DA, Schuls KF, Cates W and Tyler CW Midtrimester abortion by intraamniotic prostaglandin $F_{2a}$ safer than saline? *Obstet Gynecol* 49 612, 1977
16 Berger GS and Kerenyi TD Analysis of retained placenta associated with saline abortion clinical considerations *Am J Obstet Gynecol* 120 484, 1974
17 Grimes DA, Schulz KF, Cates W and Tyler CW Local versus general anesthesia which is safer for performing suction curettage abortions? *Am J Obstet Gynecol* 135 1030, 1979
18 Bolognese RJ and Corson SL *Interruption of Pregnancy — a Total Patient Approsch*, Williams & Wilkins, Baltimore, MD, 1975
19 Burnett LS, King TM, Atienza MF and Bell WR Intraamniotic urea as a midtrimester abortificient clinical results and serum and urinary changes *Am J Obstet Gynecol* 121 7, 1975
20 Dillon TF, Phillips LL, Risk A, Horiguchi T, Mohajer-Shojai E and Mootabar H The

efficacy of prostaglandin $F_{2a}$ in second trimester abortion Coagulation and hormonal aspects *Am J Obstet Gynecol* 118 668, 1974

21  Koplik L Disseminated intravascular coagulation after a dilation and evacuation abortion at 16 weeks gestation Paper presented at the Annual Meeting of the National Abortion Federation, Denver, Colorado, October 3, 1977

22  Stubblefield PG Alternatives for cervical dilatation work in progress In *Pregnancy Termination*, Zatuchni GI, Sciarra JJ and Speidel JJ (eds), pp 115–126 Harper & Row, Hagerstown, MD, 1979

23  Grimes DA and Cates W The comparative efficacy and safety of intraamniotic prostaglandin $F_{2a}$ and hypertonic saline for second trimester abortion *J Reprod Med* 22 248, 1979

24  Keith LG and Berger GS Prevention of Rh sensitization after abortion In *Pregnancy Termination*, Zatuchni GI, Sciarra JJ and Speidel JJ (eds), pp 294–302 Harper & Row, Hagerstown, MD, 1979

25  WHO Task Force On Sequelae of Abortion Long-term complications of induced abortion In *Pregnancy Termination* Zatuchni GI, Sciarra JJ and Spreider JJ (eds), pp 163–177 Harper & Row, Hagerstown, MD, 1979

26  Hogue CJR, Lean TH and Wood JL Long-term sequelae in dilatation and curettage versus vacuum aspiration report of an epidemiologic study in Singapore In *Pregnancy Termination*, Zatuchni GI, Sciarra JJ and Speidel JJ (eds), pp 149–155 Harper & Row, Hagerstown, MD, 1979

# 16. PREVENTION OF RHESUS (D) ISOIMMUNIZATION AFTER ABORTION

## J. Bennebroek Gravenhorst

Medical intervention can alter the course of history. According to the editor of the British Medical Journal [1] Henry the VIII was happily married to Catharine of Aragon for 19 years, and most historians agree that he would have remained married to her for the rest of his life had she borne him a son. Apart from one surviving daughter, Mary, she had several abortions and preterm labours and gave birth to five babies who died shortly after delivery.

MacLennon [2] has suggested that this horrible obstetric history could be explained by Rh immunization, if Catherine had already been sensitized by her first husband, Henry's brother Arthur. Had Rh immunoglobulin been invented, the course of English history and probably of world history might have been entirely different. The tragic deaths of Henry's future wives might have been prevented. The Church of England might not have been founded and England might have retained her American colonies [1, 2].

But it was to take many years before the prevention of haemolytic disease of the newborn became a fact.

### MECHANISM OF IMMUNIZATION

In 1940 Landsteiner and Wiener [3] found that Rh immunization was due to a foetal blood-group antigen inherited from the father, invading the maternal circulation and causing maternal immunization. A year later attention was called to the clinical significance of Rh immunization and it was shown beyond all doubt that haemolytic disease of the newborn resulted from Rh sensitization caused by transplacental haemorrhage [4, 5].

In the early forties, 45% of all Rh-immunized pregnancies resulted in intra-uterine or neonatal death [6]. Preterm delivery, amniotic fluid analysis and improved techniques in neonatal management reduced the perinatal mortality rate to 8% [7].

Although, in principle, the circulations of mother and foetus are completely separate, it is well established that foetal cells quite commonly enter the maternal circulation. Some Rh negative individuals respond with the formation of antibodies after exposure to as little as 0.1 ml of blood, others do not respond even after massive transplacental haemorrhage. In general about 70% of Rh negative individuals respond to Rh-antigenic stimulation [6, 8]. In most instances the transplacental haemorrhage is very small and bleeds of 10 ml are detected in less than 0.5% of pregnancies [8]. It is generally accepted that at least two exposures to D-antigen are needed before the development of anti-D antibodies occurs. Most foeto-maternal transfusions take place during labour and delivery, and antibody formation therefore appears very rarely during the first pregnancy (1–2%). In large control series of Rh negative women 5.2% developed antibodies within 6 months postpartum. An additional 11.5% developed antibodies in the second positive pregnancy. Thus, following a single positive pregnancy, 16.7% of Rh negative women will develop antibodies [8].

To explain the development of Rh immunization during a first pregnancy, primary sensitization due to the passage of Rh(D) positive maternal cells into a Rh(D) negative foetus has been proposed. Although there is some evidence that this mechanism may occasionally operate, the evidence is in dispute [9, 10]. Some investigators found antibodies in the blood of Rh(D) negative babies born from Rh(D) positive mothers during the first year of life [11]. The antibodies could only be demonstrated by auto-analyser techniques. These surprising findings have not been confirmed by others [12, 13]. Rh immunization of an Rh(D) negative foetus therefore is supposed to be very rare, if possible at al.

PREVENTION OF RH IMMUNIZATION

In 1961 and 1962 two independent groups of workers, Finn and associates in Liverpool [14] and Freda and Gorman in New York [15], approached the problem from different angles but arrived almost simultaneously at the same hypothesis. The Liverpool group took as a starting-point the observation that ABO incompatibility between mother and foetus offers protection against maternal Rh(D) immunization. The anti-A and anti-B isoagglutinines seem to be able to eliminate A or B cells and so prevent the production of antibodies. Experiments with Rh negative volunteers showed that chromium-51 labelled Rh positive cells could be rapidly eliminated, if anti-D serum was given shortly after the Rh positive blood injection.

Freda and co-workers based their work on the observation of Th. Smith in 1909 that diphtheria immunization by toxoid could be prevented if diphtheria antitoxin was given at the same time, in other words, that passively administered antibody suppresses the active immune response [16]. Freda and his group demonstrated in a series of experiments that Rh(D) immunization can be prevented by injecting anti-D-immunoglobulin. There are three possible mechanisms of suppressing Rh immunization [17].

1) Rh antibody may prevent the Rh antigen from reaching the germinal centres of lymph nodes and spleen where the potential immunocytes are produced.
2) Rh antibody may block or bind Rh antigenic determinants on red cell membranes so that no contact of the antigen with the surface receptors of the potential immunocytes occurs.
3) Rh antibody may have a direct suppressive effect on the potential immunocytes.

The second mechanism is the most likely one. Since anti-Rh(D) immunoglobulin came into routine use both the incidence of and mortality from haemolytic disease have fallen significantly. In Holland the incidence of new Rh-immunizations decreased from 3.5% in 1968 to 0.44% in 1978. Mortality from haemolytic disease of the newborn dropped from 147/248 000 births in 1969 to 15/175 000 births in 1979.

## ABORTION

The importance of abortion in the general picture of Rh(D) immunization has been difficult to evaluate. It appears logical to assume that placental trauma caused by therapeutic or spontaneous abortion will induce transplacental haemorrhage (T.P.H.). The incidence of T.P.H. in spontaneous abortion was estimated at about 6%. In therapeutic abortion the incidence seems to be much higher, according to some authors up to 25% [18]. Different methods of pregnancy termination such as dilatation and curettage, vacuum aspiration, abdominal hysterectomy and utus paste injection, showed no significant difference in the incidence of transplacental haemorrhage between these procedures, provided that they were carried out before 12 weeks of pregnancy [19]. The frequency of T.P.H. increases with the duration of pregnancy, and pregnancy terminations from 12 weeks onwards are reported to have a foeto-maternal transfusion rate of 16–40% [19]. Literature data on the incidence of T.P.H. in spontaneous and induced abortion show a tremendous variation. The reason for this is, among other things, the poor reproducibility of the Kleihauer method and the many modifications of that test in use.

In our own material we found transplacental haemorrhage to occur in 40% of abortions performed by aspirotomy (Beekhuizen, chapter 6) between 12 and 18 weeks of pregnancy. In these cases the foetal red cell count usually indicates a T.P.H. between 0.1 and 0.2 ml, but foeto-maternal transfusions of more than 1 ml are occasionally encountered [20]. Retrospective studies show that 3–4% of Rh negative women are immunized by an early abortion in the first pregnancy. In the Netherlands in 1978, 38 secundi gravidae developed

Rh antibodies and in 6 cases immunization was preceded by a so-called unprotected spontaneous abortion, which implies that no anti-D immunoglobulin is given.

In 1971 a WHO working group concluded that Rh immunization may occur in up to 4% of Rh negative women undergoing abortion [21]. Simonowitz [22] reported immunization rates in the next pregnancy of 3.6% in Rh negative women after unprotected abortion (11 out of 308 cases) as compared to 0.4% (13 out of 3080 cases) when 50 $\mu$g of anti-D immunoglobulin was given after abortion. Very little is known about the immunization frequency in second trimester abortion, but most investigators estimate that the risk of immunization increases proportionally with gestational age and is estimated to be 9% at three months and beyond [20, 23].

It is common practice nowadays to provide women who have a therapeutic abortion with anti-D immunoglobulin. The administration of anti-D immunoglobulin in cases of spontaneous abortion however, is often omitted and in many cases the patient's blood group is not even determined. According to Grimes [24] a candidate in the spontaneous abortion group is 18.2 times more likely not to receive anti-D immunoglobulin than a candidate in the induced abortion group [24]. In this respect the Rh prevention programme still fails in many countries [25, 26].

For early abortion a dose of 50–75 $\mu$g seems amply sufficient. In cases of second trimester abortion a dose of 200 $\mu$g is recommended [27]. The anti-D immunoglobulin should be administered within 72 hours of the antigenic stimulus, but even if this arbitrary time-limit has been inadvertently exceeded immunoprophylaxis should still be given. According to some leading investigators anti-D immunoglobulin can be given as late as 14 days after abortion, with some evidence of antibody suppression [28].

ECTOPIC PREGNANCY

Katz and Marcus [29] have pointed out that in ruptured ectopic pregnancies foetal blood is resorbed from the abdominal cavity and enters the maternal circulation [29]. Therefore, in those instances where Rh negative women are concerned, anti-D immunoglobulin should be administered.

CONCLUSIONS

Rh immunoglobulin has the potential of being-effective if given at the right time and in the proper dose. Although the incidence of Rh immunization has been considerably reduced, the lowest possible level has not yet been attained.

An important reason for this is that with induced and spontaneous abortions the utilization of anti-D immunoglobulin is still a long way off from being optimal The education of the patients and the medical profession is important in promoting a further reduction of the Rh immunization frequency All girls should have their blood typed at puberty and all Rh(D) negative women should be informed of the necessity of immunoprophylaxis after spontaneous or induced abortion Rh negative women undergoing early abortion either spontaneously or therapeutically should receive 50–75 $\mu$g anti-D immunoglobulin intramuscularly In second trimester abortion or pregnancy termination 200 $\mu$g anti-D immunoglobulin is considered to be a protective dose It should be kept in mind that the administration of anti-D immunoglobulin may have an effect on antibody suppression, even when given as late as 14 days after abortion

REFERENCES

1  MacLennan H  Gynaecologist looks at the Tudors  *Med Hist* 11  66–74, 1967
2  Editorial  Preventing Rh haemolytic disease  *Br Med J* 1  307, 1978
3  Landsteiner K and Wiener AS  Agglutinable factor in human blood recognised by immune sera for Rhesus blood  *Proc Soc Exper Biol* 43  223, 1940
4  Levine P, Katzin EM and Burnham L  Iso-immunization in pregnancy, its possible bearing on the etiology of erythroblastosis fetalis  *J Am Med Ass* 116  825–827, 1941
5  Levine P, Newark NJ, Burnham L, Englewood NJ, Katzin EM and Vogel P  The role of iso-immunization in the pathogenesis of erythroblastosis fetalis  *Am J Obstet Gynecol* 42  925–937, 1941
6  Queenan JT and Schreiner J  Practical clinical aspects of Rh-prophylaxis  *J Perinat Med* 1  223–234, 1973
7  Bevis DCA  Blood pigments in hemolytic disease of the newborn  *J Obstet Gynaecol Br Commonw* 63  68–75, 1956
8  Zipursky A  Rh hemolytic disease of the newborn, the disease eradicated by immunology  *Clin Obstet Gynecol* 20  759–772, 1977
9  Taylor JF  Sensitization of Rh negative daughters by their Rh positive mothers  *N Engl J Med* 276  547–551, 1967
10  Ramos de Almeida JH and Lino Rosado  Rh blood group of grandmother and incidence of erythroblastosis  *Arch Dis Child* 47  609–612, 1972
11  Bowen FW and Renfield M  The detection of anti D in Rh (D) negative infants born of Rh (D) positive mothers  *Pediatr Res* 10  213–215, 1976
12  Scott JR, Beer AE, Guy LR, Liesch M and Elbert G  Pathogenesis of Rh immunization in primigravidae, feto maternal versus materno fetal bleeding  *Obstet Gynecol* 49  9–14, 1977
13  Bernard B, Presley M and Candillo G  Maternal fetal haemorrhage incidence and sensitization  *Abstr Pediatr Res* 11  467, 1977
14  Finn R, Clarke CA, Donohoe WTA, McConnell RB, Sheppard PH, Lehane D and Kulke W  Experimental studies on the prevention of Rh haemolytic disease  *Br Med J* 1  1486–1490, 1961
15  Freda VJ, Gorman JG and Pollock W  Successful prevention of experimental Rh sensitization in man with an anti-Rh gammaglobulin antibody preparation  *Transfusion* 4  26–32, 1964
16  Smith T  Active immunity produced by so-called balanced or neutral mixtures of diphtheria *toxin and anti-toxin J Exp Med* 11  241–256, 1909

17  Bowman JH  Suppression of Rh-isoimmunization  A review  *Obstet Gynecol* 52  385–393, 1978

18  Matthews CD and Matthews AEB  Transplacental haemorrhage in spontaneous and induced abortion  *Lancet* 1  694–695, 1969

19  Voigt JC and Britt RP  Feto-maternal haemorrhage in therapeutic abortion  *Br Med J* 4  395–396, 1969

20  Goldman JA and Eckerling B  Prevention of Rh immunization after abortion with anti-Rh (D) immunoglobulin  *Obstet Gynecol* 40  366–370, 1972

21  WHO  Prevention of Rh sensibilization  *Wld Hlth Org Techn Rep Ses* 468  1, 1971

22  Simonovitz I  Personal communication to C Clarke  McMasters conference on prevention of Rh immunization 28–30 Sept 1977  *Vox Sang* 36  50–64, 1979

23  Freda VJ, Gorman JG, Galen RS and Treacy N  The threat of Rh immunization from abortion  *Lancet* 11  147–148, 1970

24  Grimes DA, Ross WC and Hatcher RA  Rh immunoglobulin utilization after spontaneous and induced abortion  *Obstet Gynecol* 50  261–263, 1979

25  Clarke C and Whitfield AGW  Death from Rhesus haemolytic disease in England and Wales in 1977  Accuracy of records and assessment of anti-D prophylaxis  *Br Med J* 1  1665–1669, 1979

26  Wysowski DK, Flint JW, Goldberg MF and Connell FA  Rh hemolytic disease epidemiologic surveillance in the United States, 1968 to 1975  *J Am Med Ass* 242  1376–1379, 1979

27  Keith IG and Berger GS  Prevention of Rh sensitization after abortion  *Pregnancy Termination Procedures, Safety and New Developments*, Zatuchni GI, Sciarra JJ and Speidel JJ (eds), pp 294–301  Harper & Row, Hagerstown MD, 1979

28  Samson D and Mollison PL  Effect on primary Rh immunization of delayed administration of anti Rh  *Immunology* 28  349–357, 1975

29  Katz J and Marcus RG  The risk of Rh iso-immunization in ruptured tubal pregnancy  *Br Med J* 3  667–669, 1972

# 17. CONTRACEPTION FOLLOWING SECOND TRIMESTER ABORTION

Louis G. Keith and Gary S. Berger

Women who obtain abortions in the second trimester clearly should receive thorough contraceptive counseling whether their abortion has been requested for medical or for social reasons. Since second trimester abortions take place in specialized clinics or in hospitals, these institutions are in an ideal position to direct the patient's attention to contraception. They also can provide an appropriate setting to receive family planning services as well as long-term follow-up and re-examination.

Among the advantages of using the abortion process as the starting point of contraceptive services are the following [1]:

1. Proven fertile women are easily reached.
2. Little or no self-motivation is required to request contraceptive information.
3. Active contraceptive intervention reduces the risk of immediate postabortal conception, since most women normally resume fecundity after each natal event.
4. Family planning advice may be more acceptable if given by the institution which has just supervised the successful care of a woman.
5. Proper contraception after abortion may be helpful in providing a higher standard of maternal and infant health at a later date.

Health workers desiring to provide contraceptive services to women who have undergone abortion must realize that the patterns of contraceptive behavior which preceded the abortion, i.e., either a lack of desire to use contraception or poor compliance in proper contraceptive utilization, may recur once the immediacy of the problem has been solved. This is particularly true in certain second trimester abortions where the patients have denied needing an abortion until after the first trimester or where they have had repeated abortions.

In clinical practice, women readily may agree to accept an effective contraception method prior to their abortion. Afterwards, however, the fact that the abortion procedure has been safe and comfortable may adversely affect any newly found enthusiasm for following through on contraceptive plans. Moreover, because some patients have been able to obtain their abortions freely through a system of social welfare, enthusiastic contraceptive efforts may not be constructed. Such patients may be inclined to evade any serious

*M.J.N.C. Keirse et al. (eds.), Second Trimester Pregnancy Termination. All rights reserved.*
*Copyright © 1982 Martinus Nijhoff Publishers, The Hague/Boston/London.*

and meaningful discussion of contraception, especially if they are young, unmarried or unable to pay for continuing follow-up care. This latter problem is probably more serious in the United States where medical care is generally obtained on a fee-for-service basis than it is in European countries which have more extensive social and medical welfare systems.

Whether the primary focus in the abortion procedure has been medical or social in nature, there is no room for complacency by the medical community. Patients must understand that even though present contraceptives are not 'perfect', their proper and continued utilization poses less of a threat to health than when no method is used and, in some circumstances, represents a substantial reduction in the risk to health compared to when abortion is used as the sole method of contraception [2]. The patient also must clearly understand that the likelihood of an unplanned pregnancy depends not only on the effectiveness of the contraceptive method selected and her natural level of fertility (which can be expected to decline with advancing age), but also on her adherence to the prescribed contraceptive routine.

## DEMOGRAPHIC FACTORS AFFECTING CONTRACEPTIVE USE AND ABORTION

Contraceptive use and abortion are associated phenomena in sexually active women. According to Moore-Cavar [3], international surveys of women who have had abortions indicate that these individuals were more likely to have used contraception at some prior time than women who had not had abortions. Similarly, women who had used contraception at some time were more likely to have had an abortion than women who never used contraception [3]. In spite of this association, contraceptive use in the months prior to conception among women hospitalized for complications of abortion often is low. This is true for developed as well as developing countries where access to effective contraceptives may be difficult (Table 1). On the other hand, contraceptive use increases markedly after abortion. Perhaps more importantly, the use of effective methods increases in developed as well as in developing countries, after legal and illegal abortion and after medically complicated and uncomplicated abortions. The postabortion acceptance of contraception, at least in the hospital setting, is influenced by personal characteristics such as marital status, age, parity and education on the one hand and the availability of contraceptives and the quality of counseling programs, on the other [4].

## PHYSIOLOGIC CHANGES ASSOCIATED WITH THE POSTABORTAL STATE

Considerable data exist regarding the physiological changes observed in the

Table 1 Contraceptive use before and after hospital treatment for abortion complications, selected studies 1972–1979 *

| Country | Author and year | Before abortion | | | After abortion | | |
|---|---|---|---|---|---|---|---|
| | | No interviewed | % using any method | % using effective method | No interviewed | % using any method | % using effective method |
| India | Brenner et al 1973 | 2230 | 25 | 23 | 2230 | 88 | 86 |
| Indonesia | Bernard et al 1975 | 1072 | 19 | 15 | 1057 | 30 | 24 |
| Thailand | Bernard et al 1975 | 1613 | 4 | 2 | 1463 | 47 | 44 |
| Sudan | Rushwan et al 1976 | 3263 | 10 | 10 | 2739 | 47 | 46 |
| USA | Miller 1977 | 5883 | 48 | 45 | 3518 | 93 | 85 |

* Adapted from Population Reports, Series F No 7 Table II, 1980 [4]

puerperium; similar data, however, are almost totally lacking after interruption of pregnancy in the second trimester. Most studies regarding postabortal patients have been concerned with pregnancies which were interrupted during the first trimester. In this circumstance, ovulation often returns more rapidly in the early postabortum than in the postpartum period, frequently within the first month [5]. It has been inferred that the physiologic changes observed after second trimester abortion might differ somewhat, particularly with reference to the time required for involution the uterus. Since the second trimester lasts for 12 weeks, there is opportunity for wide variation in the involution process.

*Involution of the Uterus*

By the 14th day postpartum, the uterus generally has involuted from a size of 1000 or more g to about 350 g. Similarly, by the 14th day postabortum, uteri have greatly reduced in size. Some return to their approximate prepregnancy size; others, however, remain somewhat increased in bulk for the rest of the patient's life. In all probability, the specific findings in a given patient are as dependent on individual biologic characteristics as they are on the duration of gestation.

As is the case after term delivery, three major complications may interfere with the postabortal involutionary process and restoration of the prepregnancy state of health:

1. hemorrhage from retained products of conception;
2. infection, generally related to either retained products of conception or improper abortion techniques;
3. subinvolution, related to hemorrhage and/or infection or without apparent cause.

Should one or more of these processes interfere with the postabortal involution of the uterus, the provision of adequate therapy permits the continuation of the involutionary process in the vast majority of cases.

*Lactation*

In contrast to the situation observed after first trimester abortion, patients who are farther along in pregnancy (especially after 16 gestational weeks) are more likely to experience some degree of breast engorgement and possibly even lactation. The normal physiology of lactation is based upon a gradual clearing of the steroids produced by the placenta, coincident with the appearance of spontaneous lactation triggered by pituitary hormones. During pregnancy which continues to term, estrogen and progesterone stimulate the development of the ducts and secretory alveoli. After postpartum removal of the placental tissue, the hormones derived from it are rapidly cleared from the maternal circulation and prolactin begins to influence milk secretion. With the diminished influence of the placental hormones, breast sensitivity increases dramatically. Variations in breast sensitivity are demonstrable at other times of a woman's life as well, including during the menstrual cycles of women taking oral contraceptives. It has been postulated that this phenomenon may have a key role in the initiation of the feedback cycles which maintain lactation.

It is precisely because lactation is not maintained after second trimester abortion, except in rare pathological circumstances, that prolactin begins to decline, thus permitting the appearance of LH in increasing quantities as an antecedent to the next ovulation.

The duration and degree of the lactational process after second trimester abortion varies from patient to patient, depending to an extent on the presence or absence of prior lactational experience and the gestational age of the pregnancy at the time of the abortion.

IMMEDIATE CONTRACEPTIVE POSSIBILITIES

Four methods of contraception commonly utilized after second trimester abortion are: a) sterilization, b) intrauterine devices, c) oral contraceptives, and d) barrier methods.

*Sterilization*

Prior to 1969, most second trimester abortion procedures which were combined with sterilization utilized hysterectomy or hysterotomy and tubal ligation. Since 1969, however, refinements in laparoscopic techniques have made the combination of abortion (first or second trimester) with sterilization a practical reality. The basic question which must be answered is whether complications accompanying the combined procedure of sterilization and abortion are more serious or frequent than those accompanying either procedure alone. A recent review of the world literature suggests that the question is far from settled [4]. Many of the studies used different methodologies and these are difficult to compare. Patients who undergo the combined procedure, however, should be aware of the increased likelihood of ectopic pregnancy in those cases in which sterilization fails and a woman becomes pregnant again [6]. A detailed discussion of this subject is presented by Rioux and Yuzpe (chapter 18).

*Intrauterine Devices*

Although intrauterine devices (IUDs) have been available for two decades, their use in the postabortal state has been advocated only recently. Prior to that, clinicians feared increased rates of perforation and infection. The fear of infection undoubtedly influenced the 1977 USFDA recommendation which listed septic abortion as a contraindication to IUD use and recommended a delay of at least 3 months before insertion. These assumptions have been challenged by recent research [4]. Numerous studies from a variety of locations demonstrate that routine postabortal IUD insertion does not lead to increased complications or decreased continuation rates and that the insertion of an IUD into an infected or potentially infected uterus does not lead to more morbidity or hospitalization [4]. Clearly the potential risks of IUD insertion after septic or illegal abortion must be weighed against delaying contraception. Since a high percentage (75%) of postabortal women ovulate within three weeks after their abortion, the possibility of pregnancy is real [4]. About 6% of women will conceive within 4 to 6 weeks after an abortion unless they are using effective contraception [4]. If a women is to be protected from another pregnancy, contraception must be available prior to discharge from the clinic or hospital, and immediate protection from pregnancy is the most important benefit of postabortal IUD insertion.

Although the exact mechanism of action of intrauterine devices is unknown, it is presently believed that they act by interfering with either fertilization or subsequent blastocyst implantation. Most IUDs are made of an 'inert' plastic. Some are medicated, either with copper or progesterone, both of which tend to increase the effectiveness of the device. IUDs must be inserted by trained clinicians. They are highly effective contraceptives, but like oral contraception, they also have recognized side effects. Some of these are minor, but on occasion, they can be of a serious or even fatal nature. Clinicians who prescribe intrauterine devices must recognize these facts and bring them to the attention of their patients.

Regular re-examination for patients with intrauterine devices is mandatory. Careful attention must be directed to specific complaints which may point to signs of serious problems. Initial re-examination should take place within 4 to 6 weeks after insertion. Subsequently, the patient should be seen at least once annually. Frequent examinations do not prevent complications per se, but they do lead to a total reevaluation of the patient's contraceptive choice. A complete discussion of the complications of intrauterine devices as well as practical suggestions to enhance their use has been presented by Edelman et al. [7].

*Oral Contraceptives*

Extensive commentary on oral contraceptives is beyond the scope of this chapter. Nonetheless, two points clearly must be considered as guiding principles in the prescription of these medications:

1. Properly taken, the effectiveness of oral contraceptives is unquestionably very high (virtually 100%).

2. Even under the best of circumstances, side effects occur to many users of oral contraceptives. Fortunately, the majority of side effects are not of a serious medical nature, though they may be the cause of pill discontinuation. For a small number of women, however, disease or injury associated with oral contraceptive use may be serious and could include disability or death.

The main question facing clinicians who prescribe oral contraceptives after second trimester abortion is when to start. Three possibilities exist: the same day, five days later, or after the first normal menstruation. Clearly the latter approach exposes the patient to another pregnancy. The problem with the early start (first or fifth day) is more theoretical than real. Clinicians feared that early use of the pill after abortion would predispose the patient to blood clots in a manner similar to the postpartum period. To our knowledge, however, no studies have ever demonstrated that pill use after abortion increases the incidence of blood clots.

*Initial Contraceptive Pill Selection*

Certain present or past contraindications to pill use are widely recognized. These are:
1. deep vein thrombophlebitis or thromboembolic disorders;
2. cerebral vascular or coronary artery disease;
3. known or suspected carcinoma of the breast;
4. known or suspected estrogen dependent neoplasia;
5. undiagnosed abnormal genital bleeding.
In addition, oral contraceptives are contraindicated when there is a known or suspected pregnancy.

Most of the serious side effects associated with pill use, with the possible exception of hypertension and altered glucose metabolism, are thought to be related to the estrogen content. Consequently, all women initiating oral contraceptives should be started, when feasible, on pills containing 50 $\mu$g or less of the estrogen preparation, and, with thorough counseling, those women who have already taken more than 50 $\mu$g should be prescribed a lower dosage. Side effects can be minimized by choosing a pill with the correct type and amount of progestogen. Of the 25 pill formulations currently manufactured in the United States, 20 contain 50 $\mu$g or less of ethinyl estradiol or 80 $\mu$g or less of mestranol.

*Barrier Methods*

Vaginal methods of contraception can be used immediately after abortion. They offer the possibility of serving either as an interim method until a decision is made regarding medical contraception or sterilization as a long-term method. In either case, their effectiveness has been documented in a number of studies and the rate of serious side effects is almost nil [8]. For many patients, the protective effect of the barrier methods against infection with Neisseria gonorrhea represents an added attraction [9].

Barrier methods of contraception act by preventing direct access of live sperm to the cervical os. The majority (diaphragms, foams, creams, jellies) are applied by the females. The condom is the only barrier contraceptive utilized by the male.

Barrier methods are particularly advantageous for highly motivated individuals, for those who do not have frequent coitus and when both partners have no objection to the slight inconvenience caused by these products. Of all the available contraceptive methods, only the barrier type has consistently been shown to reduce the chance of acquiring a venereal disease at the time of intercourse [10].

*Vaginal Spermicides*

A variety of contraceptive products may be placed into the vagina prior to coitus. While their physical form and consistency differ greatly, the active spermicidal ingredient is the same in most of them (nonoynol-9). Products differ primarily in the selection of the carrier base of inert chemical. When properly applied, vaginal spermicides provide contraception by physically covering the external cervical os as well as by their ability to kill sperm on contact.

Statistical data regarding the effectiveness of vaginal contraceptive products vary widely (Table 2). A more recent epidemiologic review of these data,

*Table 2.* Pregnancy rates per 100 woman-years, calculated by the Pearl Method, by contraceptive method.

| Method | Pregnancy rate | |
|---|---|---|
| | Selected clinical trial | Literature |
| Condoms | 4.10 | 6–29 |
| Creams and jellies | 6.33 | 5–36 |
| Diaphragm | 3.54 | 3–34 |
| Foam | 1.55 | 2–28 |
| Suppositories | 2.41 | 8–42 |

From Derman et al. [9].

however, has noted several possible reasons for these differences, not the least of which is study design [8]. As a class of agents, the currently available vaginal spermicides are probably slightly less effective than other barrier methods (diaphragm or condom) in which a mechanical barrier is always present and the contraceptive effect can be enhanced by the addition of a spermicidal cream or jelly [8].

The application of vaginal spermicides is generally easy. In the case of the suppository, intravaginal insertion is made by either partner, as high in the vagina as possible. Foams, jellies and creams all require the use of an applicator or plunger-like tube which permits deposition of the material at or about the level of the cervical os. Coital movements disperse these products around the cervix and vagina.

Even among individuals who prescribe vaginal contraceptive methods routinely, there is no agreement as to how long prior to intercourse these agents should be inserted. Users of vaginal products are cautioned to read the consumer directions. In some instances, application up to one hour before intercourse is permissible, but presumably the more recent the application, the more effective the spermicide. In the case of currently available suppositories, there must actually be a delay of 10 or more minutes before coitus, to allow the suppository to melt and diffuse [11]. If coitus is repeated, a reapplication of the preparation is not only desirable, but neccessary. Postcoital douching, if practiced, should be delayed for six to eight hours. Controlled studies, however, are lacking to justify the validity of this clinical advice.

*Diaphragm*

The diaphragm is a prescription barrier contraceptive in that it requires a fitting by trained clinician and thus cannot be bought 'over-the-counter' as can condoms and vaginal spermicides. Perhaps more importantly, its use in the immediate postabortal period is probably quite limited in that the fitting of a diaphragm should ideally take place when involution is complete and the vaginal canal has regained tonus, after about six weeks. Each woman must be individually fitted for her diaphragm. Fitting should be rechecked every two years in the absence of childbirth, second trimester abortion, vaginal surgery or a weight gain or loss of greater than 10 pounds. If positioned correctly, the diaphragm should not be felt by either sexual partner during coitus.

SUMMARY

The patient who has received a second trimester abortion clearly needs to be provided with a contraceptive method she can understand and use. All of the currently available methods can be used after abortion; these include sterilization, IUDs, pills and vaginal barrier methods. Patients should understand that while none of these methods is perfect, consistent and proper use of one of them will greatly reduce the chance of another unwanted pregnancy.

ACKNOWLEDGMENTS

This work was supported in part by the Charles A. Fields Medical Foundation, Ltd., Chicago, IL and the Center for the Advancement of Reproductive Health, Chapel Hill.

REFERENCES

1. Keith L, Labbock M, Petty J and Berger GS: *Postpartum and Postabortal Contraception.* Synapse Publications, Pittsburgh, PA, 1979.
2. Tietze C and Lewit S: Mortality associated with reversible methods of fertility regulation. *The Safety of Fertility Control*, Keith LG, Kent DR, Berger GS and Brittain JR (eds), pp. 42–48. Springer, New York, 1979.
3. Moore-Cavar EC: *International Inventory of Information on Induced Abortion*, p. 654. Internal Institute for Human Reproduction, New York, Columbia University, 1974.
4. Population Reports. Series F, No. 7. *Abortion in developing countries, April 1980*. Population information Program, Johns Hopkins University, Baltimore.
5. Lahteenmake P and Luukkainen T: Immediate postabortal contraception with a microdose combined preparation: suppression of pituitary and ovarian function and elimination of HCG. *Contraception* 17: 169, 1978.
6. Courey N, Horowitz A and Cunanan R: Sterilization combined with abortion. In: *Laparoscopy*, Philips JM (ed), pp. 182–186. Williams & Witkins, Baltimore, 1977.
7. Edelman D, Berger GS and Keith LG: *IUDs and their Complications.* G.K. Hall, Boston, 1979.
8. Berger GS and Jackson M: The effectiveness of over-the-counter vaginal contraceptives. In: *The Safety of Fertility Control*, Keith LG, Kent DR, Berger GS and Brittain JR (eds) pp. 159–166. Springer, New York, 1979.
9. Derman R, Keith LG and Berger GS: The role of vaginal contraceptives in preventing venereal disease and pregnancy. In: *The Safety of Fertility Control*, Keith LG, Kent DR, Berger GS and Brittain JR (eds), pp. 167–173. Springer, New York, 1979.
10. keith LG, Berger GS and Moss W: Cervical gonorrhea in women using different methods of contraception. *Am Vener Dis Assoc* 3: 17, 1976.
11. Querido L and Schnabel P: Evaluating the clinical effectiveness of patentex oval. In: *Vaginal Contraception*, Zatuchni GI, Sobrero AV, Speidel JJ and Sciarra JJ (eds) pp. 146–153. Harper & Row, Hagerstown, MD, 1979.

# 18. STERILIZATION COMBINED WITH MIDTRIMESTER ABORTION

## JACQUES E. RIOUX and A. ALBERT YUZPE

Female sterilization combined with midtrimester abortion is appropriate under certain circumstances [1]. *Sterilization* in this context refers to voluntary, female-oriented procedures resulting in permanent sterility. Obviously, male sterilization should also be discussed and considered as a viable alternative with married couples whose family is complete. The term *combined* with reference to sterilization and abortion implies that both procedures are performed at one and the same time. *Midtrimester abortion* is defined for the purpose of this presentation as any pregnancy termination performed between the twelfth and twenty-fourth week of pregnancy. Therefore, in this chapter, we will limit ourselves to the specific problems of midtrimester pregnancy termination combined with sterilization. One must realize, however, that in Canada and the United States, only 8% of abortions are performed beyond the twelfth week of gestation. Most of the cases involve younger patients whose future fertility potential must be conserved. The problem is, therefore, not overwhelming as far as numbers are concerned but serious in its implications. Indeed, 'appropriate under certain circumstances' will be the core of the discussion since it is essential to consider both why and how to combine both procedures.

WHY?

There is no absolute indication to perform a sterilization procedure concomitant with a midtrimester abortion. In fact, the only relative indication is one of convenience for the patient. The necessity for only a single anesthetic may also be considered in relative terms. Before considering the combined procedures, one must be well aware of the risks and the benefits involved. The patient and her partner should be well informed so that their decision to proceed is based upon factual knowledge and complete understanding of the benefits and risks of the procedure.

*The risks* involved in the combined procedures should not exceed the total of those for each individual procedure [2, 3]. Combined procedures may not always be ideal despite the advantages alluded to. A woman may be so distraught by the unwanted pregnancy that her decision to undergo concomitant sterilization may be more emotional than rational. There is often ambiguity surrounding the pregnancy since she has obviously procrastinated for more than two to three months before seeking medical help for a solution to the pregnancy. How rational, then, is her decision to undergo concomitant sterilization? She may feel that the abortion may be granted more easily if she also opts for sterilization as well, at least in situations where abortion committees still exist and in which their approval is necessary prior to all pregnancy terminations. The same reasons which justify the abortion may not be applicable to the sterilization, i.e. marital difficulties, contraceptive problems, etc. Medical and paramedical personnel dealing with these women should be well aware of these difficulties and, therefore, be prepared to assist her in the decision making process, at the same time making certain not to impose their own value judgements in the process.

The *benefits* of the combined procedures, as mentioned, are mainly those of convenience. The woman is already in a hospital or clinic setting. The procedures require only a single motivation which alleviates the necessity for her to return a second time for a planned interval sterilization. We sadly realize by experience that many do not return for this planned interval sterilization until they are pregnant once again and request a repeat abortion.

Even if the operating time for the combined procedures is slightly increased, it is probably still easier on the patient than a repeat anesthetic, especially if general anesthesia is employed. This, however, should not be the sole factor in deciding whether to combine the procedures.

HOW?

How should it be done? In some cases, the technique for the midtrimester abortion will dictate the route of approach for sterilization. We will successively elaborate on abdominal hysterotomy, vaginal hysterotomy, minilaparotomy, laparoscopy, culdoscopy, hysteroscopy and hysterectomy [4].

*Abdominal hysterotomy*

A conventional laparotomy for hysterotomy pregnancy termination will also allow simple and direct access to the tubes, which can then be occluded by any one of the various techniques without adding any risk to the patient.

It is not within the scope of this chapter to discuss the merits or disadvantages of hysterotomy as a means of midtrimester pregnancy termination. The technique is not even mentioned in this volume. However, should this modality be chosen, or a conventional laparotomy be indicated for any reason (uterine perforation, abdominal mass, peritonitis, etc.), the approach to the fallopian tubes is solved, and all that needs to be decided is the choice of surgical technique to achieve sterilization. In these cases, the access to the tubes being so easy, we feel that one should choose a technique with the lowest possible failure rate. It is a well known fact that the simpler methods such as the Pomeroy technique have a greater failure rate when performed in association with pregnancy as opposed to an interval sterilization [5]. For this reason, we favor either fimbriectomy, the Uchida, the Irving or the Cook techniques. Total salpingectomy may also be chosen but the increased risk of hemorrhage complications and the potential compromise of the ovarian blood supply, do not warrant this extensive procedure solely to achieve sterilization. Whatever the choice, complication rates attributable directly to the sterilization procedure should be negligible. Any complications of sterilization performed concomitant with hysterotomy should, therefore, be directly related to the laparotomy or hysterotomy alone.

## Vaginal Hysterotomy

The vaginal approach to the fallopian tubes may be chosen through either an anterior or posterior colpotomy, once the uterine contents have been evacuated by either amniotic instillation or D&E [6–8].

When *posterior colpotomy* is used, a major difficulty lies in visualizing the fallopian tubes as they lie higher or out of the true pelvis. Once they are identified, one must avoid excessive traction in attempting to deliver them into the surgical field to carry out the sterilization procedure. One can facilitate accessibility by mechanically retroverting the uterus by means of an atraumatic uterine manipulator, thus bringing the fundus closer to the incision [9].

The *anterior colpotomy* is slightly more difficult, but should be employed when there is coexistent pathology in the cul-de-sac. It is also more logical following vaginal hysterotomy. Whatever the case might be, only an experienced vaginal surgeon should undertake these procedures.

## Minilaparotomy

Minilaparotomy is quite applicable to sterilization following midtrimester abortion. This technique involves the use of an abdominal incision of 2–3 cm in length, which should be located according to the height of the fundus following uterine evacuation. At that point, the fallopian tubes may be grasped with relative ease and the sterilization procedure can be performed.

Advantages of the minilaparotomy procedure are that it:

1. Requires no extra equipment (although a few specific instruments may

facilitate the procedure);

2. Requires no specialized training in the use of sophisticated equipment;

3. May be performed under local anesthesia;

4. May be performed on an outpatient basis and prolonged hospitalization much beyond the time necessary to induce the abortion is unnecessary;

5. Requires no large capital outlay for specialized equipment;

6. May incorporate most methods of tubal occlusion.

Disadvantages are that:

1. It is more difficult to perform in the obese patient;

2. The remaining pelvic and abdominal anatomy cannot be visualized;

3. The incision scar, though small, is visible.

The technique of minilaparotomy has been described in detail in numerous publications [10, 11]. When performed at the time of midtrimester abortion, however, a few specific details should be stressed:

1. The bladder must be empty.

2. The fundus should be well palpated. Its height will vary following uterine evacuation.

3. A good, atraumatic uterine manipulator is essential to antevert the uterus adequately against the anterior abdominal wall to facilitate the choice of the site for the incision.

4. Local anesthesia is used with care, remembering always that excessive dosages may be toxic and that a known quantity may already have been used during abortion.

5. A 2–3 cm suprapubic incision is made through the skin, fat and anterior rectus fascia. An obese patient will require a larger incision and, therefore, should be operated in a hospital setting, preferably under general anesthesia.

6. The rectus muscles are separated and the posterior fascia and peritoneum incised. Care must be taken at this point to recognize any complications which may have occurred, such as incision of the bladder, bowel or uterus and repair made immediately.

7. By means of the uterine manipulator, each cornua is in turn brought into the incision and the tubes are identified, grasped and occluded.

8. Limited exploration of the pelvic viscera is then performed.

9. The abdominal wall is closed by suturing the various layers individually according to standard surgical techniques.

The greatest advantage of this procedure is the avoidance of the blind steps which are necessary in laparoscopy. The surgeon is able to observe each abdominal layer and all the structures as he or she proceeds. Hasson's open laparoscopy techniques also eliminates the blind steps of the standard laparoscopic procedure [2].

*Laparoscopy*

The laparoscopic approach to midtrimester sterilization is possible and in many ways is similar to postpartum laparoscopic sterilization [13–15].

Certain advantages exist with this method and include the following:

1. The procedure may be performed on an outpatient basis under neuroleptanalgesia, local, regional or general anesthesia [16].

2. Minimal postoperative recuperation time is necessary.

3. An overall assessment of pelvic and abdominal structures is possible at the same time.

4. The development of mechanical occlusive devices and bipolar electrocoagulation has virtually eliminated electrosurgical injury to viscera.

The disadvantages include:

1. Specialized training is essential [17].

2. Equipment is expensive, fragile and may be difficult to maintain under certain circumstances.

3. Because of its larger size, the uterus can be traumatized by the pneumoperitoneum needle and/or trocar. Fortunately, these can be recognized by direct evaluation and a subsequent course of management decided upon.

4. Increased and occassionally extreme vascularity in the mesosalpinx and the broad ligament makes the risk of hemorrhagic complications associated with the actual sterilization greater.

In the hands of the experienced laparoscopist the procedure carries only a slightly greater risk of complications, provided very strict criteria are followed:

1. The Verres needle should be introduced only enough to penetrate the peritoneum. The abdominal wall should be well elevated and the needle aimed vertically [18]. Alternative sites of insufflation may include the left subcostal area or the cul-de-sac.

2. To avoid a blind abdominal penetration by the sharp pneumoperitoneum needle or trocar, the 'open laparoscopy' technique developed by Hasson is very useful, if not essential [12].

3. The trocar is likewise introduced superficially.

4. If the double puncture technique is used, the second puncture site must be in a position which enables adequate mobility, i.e. higher and/or more lateral than usual.

5. When diathermy is utilized, electrocoagulation without cutting or resecting is preferable [19], and bipolar forceps [20] should always be used since the bowel will generally be in closer proximity to the enlarged uterus.

6. When a mechanical occlusion technique is used, one should be aware

that, if the tube is too thick or edematous, the Falope ring should not be used, and when the Hulka clip is employed, the surgeon must be certain that the entire width of the tube is enclosed in the jaws of the clip.

Failure rates following laparoscopic sterilization combined with midtrimester abortion are not available from the current literature. Theoretically, they should parallel those for other techniques, i.e. be slightly higher than when performed in the interval state [21].

*Culdoscopy*

With the increase in popularity of laparoscopic sterilization, the interest in performing and teaching culdoscopy has decreased markedly in North America, as well as in other parts of the world [22]. Indeed, very few programs of female sterilization are based on its use. Culdoscopy shares one disadvantage with laparoscopy, i.e. the delicate and expensive instrumentation coupled with the specialized surgical training necessary to perform the procedure. At the same time, culdoscopy has very few of the advantages. Patient positioning during the procedure has also resulted in less than enthusiastic responses from women operated under local anesthesia. Furthermore, the procedure is difficult to perform when the uterus is enlarged, although the tubes can still be fairly well visualized by this procedure following uterine evacuation. The choice of the obstructing technique is limited to the bipolar electrocoagulation, the Falope ring or the clip.

*Hysteroscopy*

Hysteroscopy can be performed during the post abortum period, but it becomes quite an accomplishment when the cavity is visualized. It would be difficult and often impossible to identify the ostia. Even then, in spite of absolute identification, the failure rates reported are far too high to be acceptable. In the pregnant state these would presumably be even higher [22].

*Hysterectomy*

Vaginal or abdominal hysterectomy for the sole purpose of achieving sterilization and abortion should be discouraged. Lesser combined procedures are available and should be chosen when there is no specific gynecologic pathology that would require immediate or possible future hysterectomy. It seems logical that indications for performing hysterectomy for sterilization and abortion be limited to the following specific indications:

1. Gynecologic pathology
    a) cervical carcinoma in situ
    b) menorrhagia and/or metrorrhagia
    c) prolapse of the uterus with or without urinary incontinence
    d) uterine fibroids
    e) chronic pelvic inflammatory disease
    f) endometriosis
    g) severe dysmenorrhea
    h) dyspareunia.
2. Previous failed sterilization (fear or recurrence).
3. Cancer phobia (strong family history).
4. Strong desire to avoid menstruation.

When the *vaginal approach* [23–25] is chosen, it should decrease operating time and postoperative morbidity, including ileus, atelectasis, adhesion formation, pain and length of hospital stay. Depending on the patient's parity, amount of pelvic relaxation and gestational age, initial uterine evacuation may not be necessary as this results in decreased loss blood. The procedure is somewhat facilitated because the tissue planes are generally easily established in the gravid state. Because of the increased vascularity, double ligatures for all vascular pedicles are recommended. Prophylactic antibiotics are highly recommended to decrease postoperative febrile morbidity.

Sometimes the *abdominal approach* [24, 25] has to be used:
1. advanced pregnancy (over 15 weeks),
2. large uterine fibroids,
3. coexisting ovarian mass,
4. extrauterine pelvic mass,
5. endometriosis,
6. pelvic inflammatory disease,
7. previous multiple cesarean sections,
8. lack of pelvic relaxation.

It may be necessary to evacuate the uterus via a hysterotomy to decrease uterine mass, but this results in increased operative loss of blood. Ureters should be identified and isolated. Double ligation of vascular pedicles is also employed. Prophylactic antibiotics are not required unless there is coexisting pelvic inflammatory disease.

CONCLUSION

Sterilization can be safely combined with midtrimester abortion. Each individual case must, however, be thoroughly evaluated first in order to ascertain that the benefits of the procedure chosen outweigh the risks.

REFERENCES

1. Yuzpe AA and Rioux JE: Pregnancy termination combined with sterilization. In: *Pregnancy Termination: Procedures, Safety and New Developments*. Zatuchni GI, Sciarra JJ and Speidel JJ (eds), pp. 312–322. Harper & Row, Hagerstown, 1979.
2. Cheng MCE and Rochat RW: The safety of combined abortion-sterilization procedure. *Am J Obstet Gynecol* 129: 548–552, 1977.
3. Edstrom KGD: The relative risks of sterilization alone and in combination with abortion. *Bull WHO* 52: 141–148, 1975.
4. Yuzpe AA: Choosing a sterilization procedure: laparoscopic tubal sterilization. *H Reprod Med* 15: 119–122, 1975.
5. Garb AE: A review of tubal sterilization failures. *Obstet Gynecol Surv* 12: 291–305, 1957.
6. Collins JA, Allen HH and Yuzpe AA: Outpatient management of first trimester therapeutic abortion with and without tubal ligation. *Can Med Assoc J* 106: 1077–1080, 1972.
7. Morris JA: Therapeutic abortion and concurrent vaginal tubal ligation. *Obstet Gynecol* 44: 144–148, 1974.
8. Yuzpe AA, Allen HH and Collins JA: Tubal sterilization: new concepts methodology, postoperative management and follow-up of 2934 cases. *Can Med Assoc J* 107: 115, 1972.
9. Yuzpe AA, Anderson RJ, Cohen NP and West JL: A review of 1035 tubal sterilizations by posterior colpotomy under local anesthesia or by laparoscopy. *J Reprod Med* 13: 106–109, 1974.
10. Osathanondh V: Supra mini-laparotomy, uterine elevation: simple, inexpensive and outpatient procedure for interval female sterilization. *Contraception* 10: 251, 1974.
11. Penfield J: Minilaparotomy, in press.
12. Hasson H: Open laparoscopy. In *Laparoscopy*, Philips JM. (ed) pp. 145—149. Williams & Wilkins, Baltimore, 1977.
13. Cunahan RG and Courey NG: Combined laparoscopic sterilization and. pregnancy termination. II. Further experiences with a larger series of patients. *J Reprod Med* 13: 204–205, 1974.
14. Keith L and Houser KT: Puerperal sterilization. In: *Laparoscopy*, Philips JM (ed.) pp. 187–190. Williams & Wilkins, Baltimore, 1977.
15. Whitson LG, Ballard CA and Israel A.: Laparoscopic tubal sterilization coincidental with therapeutic abortion by suction curettage. *Obstet Gynecol* 41: 677'680, 1973.
16. Fisburne J jr. Keith L: Anesthesia for laparoscopy. In: *Laparoscopy*, Philips JM (ed), pp. 69–85. Williams & Wilkins, Baltimore, 1977
17. Rioux JE, Quesnel G, Blanchet J, Villa J, Turmel J and Dupont P: Laparoscopie: stérilisation tubaire: étude de 1000 cas et évaluation globale de la méthode. *Union Méd Can* 102: 1865, 1973.
18. Shepard MK: Female contraceptive sterilization. *Obstet Gynecol Survey* 29: 739—787, 1974.
19. Yuzpe AA, Rioux JE, Loffer FD and Pent D: Laparoscopic tubal sterilization by the 'burn only' technic. *Obstet Gynecol* 49: 106–109, 1977.
20. Rioux JE and Cloutier D: A new bipolar instrument for laparoscopic tubal sterilization. *Am J Obstet Gynecol* 119: 737, 1974.
21. Philips J, Hulka B, Hulka J, Keith D and Keith L: Survey of laparoscopy 1971–1975. In: *Laparoscopy*, Philips JM (ed), pp. 343–352. Williams & Wilkins, Baltimore, 1977.
22. Rioux JE and Yuzpe AA: Evaluation of female sterilization procedures. *Current Problems in Obsetrics and Gynecology*, vol. 11, No. 9, Year Book Medical Publishers, Chicago, 1979.
23. Ballard CA: Therapeutic abortion and sterilization by vaginal hysterectomy. *Am J Obstet Gynecol* 118: 891–896, 1974.
24. Kreutner AK: Hysterectomy for pregnancy termination and sterilization. In: *Pregnancy Termination: Procedures, Safety and New Developments*. Zatuchni GI, Sciarra JJ and Speidel JJ (eds). pp. 323–332. Harper & Row, Hagerstown, MD, 1979.
25. Scott JS: Sterilization by hysterectomy. *Int Plann Parent Fed Med Bull* 12: 1–2, 1978.

## 19. SOMATIC SEQUELAE AND FUTURE REPRODUCTION AFTER PREGNANCY TERMINATION

### Carol J. Rowland Hogue

A decision to choose one second trimester termination method or another should be based on several factors, not the least of which is the potential impact of the termination on future reproductive potential. While one might assume that the method that produces fewest immediate complications also results in the fewest long-range effects, this assumption may not be valid. It would make sense that the procedure with least trauma would be associated with the fewest long-range problems, but this assumption needs to be examined empirically for several reasons. Firstly, damage to the reproductive system may not be immediately observable. Secondly, somatic sequelae may occur in the absence of immediate sequelae. Thirdly, when termination procedures are compared with respect to relative safety, immediate complications are often lumped together as 'major' or 'minor'. For example, when prostaglandin $F_{2\alpha}$ was compared with saline for induction of abortion at 13–24 menstrual weeks gestation in the JPSA/CDC study conducted in the United States from 1971 through 1975, operative treatments of complications were combined in the analysis [1]. These included laparotomy, hysterotomy, and hysterectomy. Combining these operative procedures, the authors concluded that prostaglandins were about five times more likely to produce serious complications requiring operative treatment. It is apparent, however, that if the complication required hysterectomy rather than either hysterotomy or laparotomy, the resultant effect on future reproduction would be profoundly different. Thus, from this report it is not possible to tell which procedure would produce the least effect on future reproduction.

For the resons listed above, one cannot rely on relative rates of immediate complications to compare second trimester methods with respect to somatic sequelae and future reproduction. Direct observation of long-term complications is called for. Somatic sequelae which have been examined to some extent following all induced abortions or following first trimester procedures include menstrual irregularities, secondary infertility, ectopic pregnancies, complications of pregnancy, subsequent fetal loss, low birth weight, shortened gestation, and infant mortality (for reviews, see 2, 3). All of these problems should also be studied following second trimester terminations.

To date, such necessary studies of late sequelae of second trimester procedures have been very meager, despite the fact that the earliest investigations of late sequelae were of second trimester abortions; see Lindahl [4] for a careful longitudinal study of vaginal hysterotomy, a procedure no longer much used. More recent epidemiological studies involving comparison groups have limited investigation to the first trimester, since most series of abortion histories have contained too few cases of second trimester procedures to justify analysis [5, 6] or have been unable to obtain the necessary information on abortion procedure to include that analysis in their study [2, 7].

There is virtually no information regarding the incidence of secondary infertility subsequent to second trimester abortions. Evidence from follow-up studies of first trimester abortions suggests that women who have terminated their first pregnancies by abortion may actually be more fertile than counterparts who carry their first pregnancy to term. This is illustrated in Fig. 1 which shows the probability of remaining in a non-pregnant state by months since ceasing contraception. For example, after nine months of unprotected intercourse, 66% of the first pregnancy aborters had conceived, but only 42% of the first pregnancy deliverers had become pregnant again. It may be that unusually fertile women are more likely to be faced with an unwanted pregnancy which they terminate with abortion, while less fertile, sexually active women do not become pregnant under similar circumstances [8]. Whether

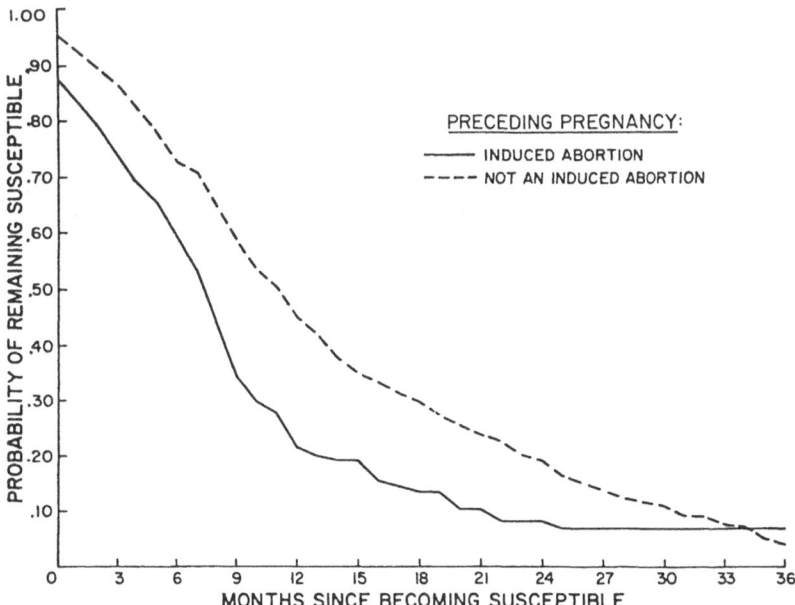

*Fig. 1.* Life table probabilities of remaining susceptible to pregnancy (i.e., not pregnant while exposed) by outcome of the immediately preceding pregnancy, for married non-contracepting women in Skopje, Yugoslavia, sample (From Hogue et al. [8]).

*Table 1.* Some particulars of the termination procedure of potential impact on somatic sequelae.

| |
| --- |
| Method of termination |
| Immediate complications |
| Degree of dilatation, if dilated |
| Method of dilatation |
| Exact gestation at termination |

second trimester procedures follow this pattern is open to question, since the procedures themselves may exert an adverse effect on subsequent fertility. This is a question which should be answered, for many women seeking second trimester abortions will wish to have a child some time in the future.

Second trimester procedures may differ in their impact on subsequent fertility or fertility-related problems. As listed in Table 1, several features of the procedure may affect future reproduction and/or somatic sequelae. These include method of termination, type of immediate complications, degree of dilatation (if dilated), method of dilatation, and exact gestation at termination. Fragmentary information exists concerning three of these aspects, namely type of procedure, existence of immediate complications, and degree of dilatation. Briefly, let us review this information.

PROCEDURE-SPECIFIC SEQUELAE

One study exclusively of saline instillation was reported by Borenstein et al. [9] in 1979. Pregnancies of each of 213 women had been aborted by instillation of a solution of 30% saline into the amniotic sac. No oxytocin was administered. Curettage completed the procedure in more than 85% of the cases. These procedures were performed over a period of 22 years, beginning in 1955, at the Kaplan Hospital in Rehovot, Israel. When an attempt to follow the women was made in the late 1970s, 103 of the 213 were contacted.

A feature of this study, which is a fairly common finding for second trimester studies, is that 66% of the abortions had been performed because of medical problems, such as death in utero or maternal rubella. Somewhat surprising was that gestations exceeded the twenty-sixth week for almost one-fourth of the pregnancies.

Women were given gynecological examinations, and their subsequent pregnancy history was determined. Three conditions were discovered which could be attributed to the procedure: hydrosalpinx, cervical incompetence, and intrauterine adhesions. One of two cases of secondary infertility could have been due to the procedure as well. Of the 68 women who reported at least one subsequent conception, only two had experienced a spontaneous abortion (Table 2). This very low rate could be due to underreporting, but it is not

Table 2. Pregnancies following second trimester procedures by type of procedure.

| Termination procedure | Number of pregnancies | Spontaneous abortions | | Pre-term deliveries | Full-term deliveries |
|---|---|---|---|---|---|
| | | < 12 wks | ≥ 12 wks | | |
| *Saline Instillation* | | | | | |
| Borestein [9] | 68 | —————— 2 —————— | | * —————— | 66 —————— |
| Daling and Emanuel [10] | 30 | ——————————————— 3 | | | 27 |
| Slater et al. [11] | 18 | ——————————————— 1 | | | 17 |
| *Dilatation and Evacuation* | | | | | |
| Peterson [12] | 242 | —————— 34 —————— 35 | | | 173 |
| Hanson [13] | 11 | ——————————————— 0 | | | 11 |
| Hogue et al. (unpublished) | | | | | |
| D&C | 18 | —————— 3 —————— 3 | | | 12 |
| D&E | 16 | —————— 2 —————— 1 | | | 13 |
| Obel [14] | 67 | | | 9 | 58 |
| *Prostaglandins $PGE_2$ or $PGF_{2\alpha}$* | | | | | |
| MacKenzie and Hillier [15]+ | 144 | 12 (8.4)§ | 7 (2.4) | 4 6.5) | 121 (124.5) |

* Dashes indicate that information was unavailable.
+ 92% of abortions were performed after the twelfth week of gestation.
§ Expected number based on a comparison group of similar social class but lower average parity and higher average age.

possible to examine this potential bias since no comparison group was utilized in the study.

Two other studies have reports of pregnancies following saline instillations. One [10] was a record review of 590 women who reported a previous induced abortion among a total of 4896 women treated for pregnancy in Seattle, Washington from 1972 through 1976. Barely 5% of the abortions had been performed with saline instillation, and 10% of these were born prematurely. Because of the small number, the rate of prematurity was not significantly different from the rate for all women with previous induced abortion nor from the control prematurity rate. Similarly, the low birth weight rate among the 18 women terminated by saline was not significantly different from the rate experienced by all aborted women who were studied by means of record linkage at the Hebrew University-Hadassah Medical School from 1967 through 1976 [11].

In sum, only 118 pregnancies following saline instillation for second tri-mester termination of pregnancy have been reported in the medical literature. This number is far too small to provide definitive answers to the questions of long-term complications. Furthermore, half of the pregnancies were reported in studies of all termination procedures, and these studies included a fairly large number of pregnancies for which the previous abortion could not be classified according to termination procedure. It is possible that reports from those studies are biased by selective reporting of procedures.

Three times as many pregnancy histories have been reported following dilatation and evacuation procedures as following saline inductions. Two-thirds of these are from Peterson's series [12] while the remainder are distributed among three other studies [13, 14, Hogue et al., unpublished]. While Hanson's small series [13] includes no adverse pregnancy outcome, the remaining series report prematurity rates ranging from 13 to 17%, and spontaneous abortion rates ranging from 14 to 15%. The relative uniformity of these reports which span ethnic, recial, and socioeconomic differences of a vast nature may be coincidental or actual. It is not possible to say whether they represent a true picture of the experience of women following pregnancies terminated by dilatation and evacuation however, because the largest series contains no controls and the other series, while controlled (in Singapore by comparison with pregnancies following no induced abortion and with those following first trimester procedures, and in Denmark by comparison with pregnancies following other termination procedures), are far too small to provide reliable estimates.

Only one study of the long-term effects of prostaglandin-induced abortions has been reported [15]. In a semi-controlled study of 144 pregnancies following extra-amniotic (n = 94) or intra-amniotic (n = 50) administration of prostaglandins, 16% of the subsequent pregnancies were spontaneously aborted or delivered prematurely. A comparison group experienced an adverse pregnancy rate of 13.5%, but these rates are not strictly comparable since the comparison group was slightly older and of lower parity, and rates were not standardized by age and parity. Furthermore, pregnancy histories were obtained in a different fashion for each group; the control group's histories were obtained solely through maternity records while the abortion series' records came from questionnaires. This difference could have produced relative underreporting of first trimester spontaneous abortions for the comparison series.

COMPLICATION-SPECIFIC SEQUELAE

If information regarding the effect of particular procedures on subsequent reproduction is lacking, information about the effect of immediate complications on the rate of long-term complications is almost non-existent. Obel's study in Denmark [14] sheds some light on the effect of immediate complications of vacuum aspiration. Table 3 summarizes his findings on this

*Table 3.* Percentage low birth weight by termination procedure, Denmark 1974–1975 (based on data from Obel [14]).

| | Number of pregnancies | Number weighing ≤ 2500 g | Percentage weighting ≤ 2500 g |
|---|---|---|---|
| Vacuum aspiration (VA) with no additional curettage | 394 | 23 | 5.8 |
| Vacuum aspiration (VA) complicated with recurettage | 21 | 5 | 23.8 |
| Dilatation and curettage* (D&C) | 45 | 3 | 6.7 |
| Other methods+ | 62 | 6 | 9.7 |

\* 60% were dilated > 12 mm
+ Saline instillation (n = 25), intra-amniotic prostaglandins (n = 10), extra-amniotic prostaglandins (n = 6), hysterotomy (n = 4), other (n = 17).

subject. Of 415 pregnancies terminated by vacuum aspiration, 21 (5%) required recurettage. Those women subsequently experienced a highly significant, fourfold rise in rate of low birth weight. These abortions were both first and second trimester procedures, so the results cannot be exactly extrapolated to the second trimester. Also, the degree of dilatation and type of curettage employed are not reported. That they differ from traditional D&C may be inferred from the subsequent pregnancy histories. Pregnancies following D&C had a significant, 3.55 times lower rate of low birth weight than those following vacuum aspiration with recurettage.

DILATATION-SPECIFIC SEQUELAE.

There is considerable concern about the long-range effects of dilating the pregnant cervix by more than 12 mm. Evidence supporting this concern may be found in such studies as those by Johnstone et al. [16], Obel [14] and Slater et al. [11]. Johnstone et al. [16] discovered that dilatation of 12 mm or more was related to enlarged cervical diameter on follow-up examination. The study by Slater et al. [11], including information on degree of dilatation of the previous abortion for 63 subsequently pregnant women, found increased rates of low birth weight for women who had been dilated by 12 mm or more. This association was not significant, however, due to the small numbers in the groups being compared. Results of the Obel study [14] are summarized in Table 4. Pregnancies terminated by vacuum aspiration which involved dilatation greater than 12 mm were 2.5 times more likely to be followed by low birth weight deliveries than were pregnancies terminated by vacuum aspi-

*Table 4.* Percentage low birth weight by degree of dilatation, Denmark 1974–1975 (based on data from Obel [14]).

|  | Number of pregnancies | Number weighing ≤2500 g | Percentage weighing ≤2500 g |
|---|---|---|---|
| VA dilated ≤12 mm* | 337 | 18 | 5.3 |
| D&C (60% > 12 mm) | 45 | 3 | 6.7 |
| VA dilated >12 mm* | 67 | 9 | 13.4 |

\* An unknown number were complicated by recurettage.

ration with dilatation of 12 mm or less. This finding, which is statistically significant, must be considered in light of the fact that an unknown number of vacuum aspiration procedures in each category of dilatation were complicated by recurettage. It is possible that the recurettage was the precipitating factor rather than the initial degree of dilatation. It is interesting that the D&C procedures, 60% of which involved dilatation greater than 12 mm, had a subsequent low birth weight rate more similar to the less-dilated vacuum aspiration procedures.

INDIVIDUAL RISK-SPECIFIC SEQUELAE.

A woman whose pregnancy is aborted in the second trimester may have individual characteristics which would place her in a high-risk category for subsequent pregnancy complications, irrespective of the abortion being performed. Most abortions based on medical indications occur in the second trimester. Some of these conditions may persist to plague future pregnancies which are attempted to be carried to term. Women whose second trimester abortions are performed on the basis of social indications often comprise a high-risk group as well, because of sociodemographic correlates such as maternal age, parity, economic status, marital status, and failure to seek care in the first trimester. Table 5 lists some, but by no means all, of the personal characteristics which may affect the probability of an adverse outcome of a subsequent pregnancy. Any such confounding variables should be examined for their effect on an association between second trimester procedure and somatic sequelae.

As an example of the importance of these personal characteristics, consider the age when the second trimester abortion occurs. As can be seen in Table 6, in most countries for which there is information on age and gestation at termination, around 40% of second trimester abortions are performed on teenagers or pre-teenagers. For the very young, pregnancy carried to term is risky. If they are able to postpone their first birth through abortion, they may

*Table 5.* Personal characteristics of potential impact on somatic sequelae.

Medical indication (if any) for termination
Previous pregnancy history
Age at termination
Socio-economic status
Interval to subsequent conception
Marital status at time of subsequent event
Smoking during subsequent pregnancy
Alcohol consumption during subsequent pregnancy
Other risk factors during subsequent pregnancy

actually be reducing this risk [10]. Should studies of these women reveal no difference in adverse outcome rates between primigravid teens and postabortion nulliparous teens, matched for age at delivery, this result could really signal lower risk to those who are postabortion, since second births to teens are at higher risk than are first births [18, 19].

SUGGESTIONS FOR FUTURE RESEARCH

Are women who obtain a second trimester abortion trading the alleviation of emergent problems for the pain of future somatic problems? If medical indications such as rubella or intrauterine death dictate the abortion, then there is no doubt that present benefit outweighs potential future risk. Also, if no further reproduction is contemplated, then only potential somatic sequelae such as menstrual irregularities should be considered when weighing the costs of the procedure against its benefits. There is no clearcut statement of risks to future reproduction for any of the second trimester procedures. Cost–benefit analysis for the young, nulliparous patient is impossible to calculate at present. Further investigations are indicated which will seek answers to these questions.

*Table 6.* Estimated percentage of distribution of second trimester abortions by age, selected areas and years.*

| Area | Aged ≤ 19 | Aged ≥ 20 |
|------|-----------|-----------|
| Canada, 1976 | 44 | 56 |
| England and Wales, 1975[+] | 37 | 63 |
| Hungary, 1975 | 45 | 55 |
| Japan, 1977 | 10 | 90 |
| Sweden, 1976 | 36 | 64 |
| United States, 1972–75 | 45 | 55 |

* The proportions were estimated using data from Tietze [17].
[+] Residents only.

Future studies should deal with several problems inherent in this field of research Firstly, since second trimester procedures are often performed on the basis of medical rather than social indications, it is crucial that analysts control for previous risk status when comparing subsequent outcomes Secondly, sufficient information about patients' personal risk factors should be collected Thirdly, sufficient information about the termination procedure must be gathered to enable investigation of various aspects of the procedure with respect to the impact of each aspect on future reproduction Fourthly, it is important to ensure a high degree of follow-up of a large group of women so that results will be stable and representative of the population sample Fifthly, comparison groups must be followed as well Depending on the research question, one of several groups might be appropriate, such as women who were aborted in the first trimester, women not aborted who are of equivalent parity, and women not aborted who are of equivalent gravidity

With careful attention to such details, it is possible to carry out good research of the long-term complications of second trimester pregnancy termination The importance of such research cannot be overemphasized in the ongoing discussion of the relative safety of different abortion procedures

## REFERENCES

1  Grimes DA, Schulz KF, Cates W, Jr and Tyler CW, Jr  Methods of midtrimester abortion which is safest? *Int J Gynaecol Obstet* 15  184–188, 1977
2  Maine D  Does abortion affect later pregnancies? *Int Fam Plann Perspect* 5  22–25, 1979
3  Hogue CJ  Reproduction after first trimester induced abortion  *The Safety of Fertility Control*, Keith LG, Kent DR, Berger GS and Brittain JR (eds), pp 220–232  Springer, New York, 1980
4  Lindahl J  *Somatic Complications following Legal Abortions*  Scandanavian University Books, Stockholm, 1959
5  Hogue CJF  Low birth weight subsequent to induced abortion in a historical prospective study of 948 women in Skopje, Yugoslavia  *Am J Obstet Gynecol* 123  675–681, 1975
6  WHO Task Force on the Sequelae of Abortion  Gestation, birthweight, and spontaneous abortion in pregnancy after induced abortion  *Lancet* 1  142–145, 1979
7  Harlap S, Shiono P, Ramcharan S, et al  A prospective study of spontaneous fetal losses following induced abortion  *N Eng J Med* 301  677–681, 1979
8  Hogue CJ, Schoenfelder JR, Gesler WM and Shachtman RH  The interactive effects of induced abortion, interpregnancy interval and contraceptive use on subsequent pregnancy outcome  *Am J Epidemiol* 107  15–26, 1978
9  Borenstein R, Ashkenazy M and Lancet M  Early complications and late sequelae of hypertonic saline induction  Presented at the Fifth European Congress on Sterility and Fertility Venice, Italy, 1979  Reported in *Ob-Gyn News*, p 46, March 1, 1979
10  Daling JR and Emanuel I  Induced abortion and subsequent outcome of pregnancy in a series of American women  *N Eng J Med* 297  1241–1245, 1977
11  Slater PE, Davies AM and Harlap S  The effect of method of abortion on the outcome of subsequent pregnancy  *J Reprod Med* 26  123–138, 1981
12  Peterson WF  Dilatation and evacuation  patient evaluation and surgical techniques  Presented at the Workshop and Postgraduate Course on Pregnancy Termination Procedures,

Safety, and New Developments. Nassau, Bahamas, May 23–26, 1978.

13. Hanson M: D&E midtrimester abortion. Presented at the 16th Annual Meeting of the Association of Planned Parenthood Physicians. San Diego, CA, October 26, 1978.

14. Obel E: Pregnancy complications following legally induced abortion with special reference to abortion technique. *Acta obstet gynaecol Scand* 58: 147–153, 1979.

15. Mackenzie IZ and Hillier K: Prostaglandin-induced abortion and outcome of subsequent pregnancies: a prospective controlled study. *Br Med J* 2: 1114–1117, 1977.

16. Johnstone FD, Beard RJ, Boyd IE et al.: Cervical diameter after suction termination of pregnancy. *Br Med J* 1: 68–69, 1976.

17. Tietze C: *Induced Abortion: 1979* (3rd edn). The Population Council, New York, 1979.

18. Jekel JF, Harison JT, Bancroft DRE, et al.: A comparison of the health of index and subsequent babies born to school age mothers. *Am J Public Health* 65: 370–374, 1975.

19. United States Department of Health, Education and Welfare: Weight at birth and survival of the newborn by age of mother and total-birth order. *Vital Health Stat* 21: 33–39, 1965.

## 20. PSYCHOSOCIAL ASPECTS OF PREGNANCY TERMINATION

E.V. VAN HALL

For a woman faced with an unwanted pregnancy three options are available:
1. termination of pregnancy,
2. acceptance of pregnancy and child,
3. acceptance of pregnancy but not of the child (adoption).

It is difficult to discuss the psychosocial aspects of pregnancy termination without taking into account the latter two options. In fact one may ask oneself whether the early and late emotional reactions to a wanted pregnancy should not be taken into consideration as well.

Unlike other difficult and far-reaching decisions in life (e.g. marriage, divorce, parenthood, sterilization), the decision whether or not to terminate an unwanted pregnancy is rather unique because it has to be made in a critical situation within a limited period of time. Another unique aspect of the decision-making process is that acceptance of the pregnancy is irreversible and involves the future life of both the parent and the unborn child, whereas termination of the pregnancy allows the possibility of deciding in favour of a wanted pregnancy at another stage of life.

To review the literature on this subject and draw general conclusions is not an easy task, because the studies have been conducted and published at different points of time during a period in which attitudes towards abortion have changed considerably. It is clear by now that the occurrence of emotional reactions after abortion is closely related to the social acceptance of contraception in general and abortion in particular within society at large and in the environment of the woman in question. Another difficulty in reviewing the literature on this subject is that much of this literature is plagued by limited research methodology and by the intrusion of an ideological bias reflecting the researchers views on the morality of abortion and on the proper role of women in society [1]. Hence, most of the studies which have reported a high rate of adverse psychological sequelae of abortion are based on impressionistic reports of a few cases rather than on data acquired by systematic research on larger groups [1, 2]. Finally, interpretation of the literature is hampered by the fact that only a few studies also consider the consequences of denial of abortion and there are no studies either on the early and late emotional reactions to having placed the child for adoption or on the psychosocial follow-up of women who did not even consider abortion but accepted their unwanted pregnancy for legal, social or religious reasons.

Despite these reservations an attempt will be made to provide some information on the psychological effects of pregnancy termination. It should be noted that this information is based on relatively recent, and predominantly American, literature ('post-liberalization studies'). This choice of literature also reflects the author's personal attitude towards the problem of unwanted pregnancy.

PSYCHOSOCIAL ASPECTS OF PREGNANCY TERMINATION IN GENERAL

Two thorough and comprehensive reviews should be mentioned in this context. Illsley and Hall [2] published an extensive review of the issues and the necessary research needed on the psychosocial aspects of abortion. They conclude that, where careful pre- and postabortion assessments are made, psychological benefit commonly results, and serious adverse emotional sequelae are rare. On the other hand, the outcome of refused abortion seems to be less satisfactory, with regrets and distress frequently occuring. Although many women who are refused abortion adjust to their situation and grow to love their child, about half of them would still have preferred abortion, while a large minority suffer considerable distress, and a small minority develop severe mental disturbance. David [3] also reviewed the literature on this subject and concludes that legally induced abortion does not carry a significant risk of psychiatric trauma and that, whatever psychological risk exists this is less than that associated with carrying a pregnancy to term. For the vast majority of women abortion engenders a sense of relief and represents a maturing experience of successfully coping with a critical situation. Adler [4] analysed postabortion emotional responses in 95 women. She concludes that the predominant emotional responses to abortion are happiness and relief, but that these emotions may often be combined with mild to moderate feelings of guilt, regret and depression. Finally, Osofsky et al. [5], evaluating the psychological effects of abortion, conclude that for most women, abortion appears to be accompanied by few, if any, negative psychological sequelae. More often abortion appears to lead to individual growth and resolution of problems.

PSYCHOSOCIAL ASPECTS OF SECOND TRIMESTER PREGNANCY TERMINATION

Very few studies have been published on this specific aspect of abortion. As it is likely that the emotional value of a pregnancy increases with the length of gestation, it could be expected that adverse emotional reactions would occur more frequently after late- than after early-induced abortion [6]. It should be borne in mind, however, that women who delay the decision of abortion until midtrimester represent a special population (Ketting, chapter 2). Although there appears to be little, if any, difference in psychological characteristics between women who opt for early or late abortion, and those who delay the decision for abortion until the second trimester of pregnancy tend to evade facing the reality of both the pregnancy and the abortion [7]. On the average they are younger, less educated, more frequently single and less often employed [8]. The delay in seeking or obtaining abortion is most often due to intrinsic factors of pregnancy-denial, ambivalence and fear, although physician-induced delays and delays due to laboratory errors in pregnancy diagnosis are unacceptably frequent [9]. Finally, it should be realized that the techniques used for late pregnancy termination are more radical and hazardous (as compared to vacuum aspiration) and can thus contribute to a higher incidence of immediate post-abortion emotional reactions.

CONCLUSIONS

In conclusion it can be stated that the decision to terminate an unwanted pregnancy is often difficult and emotionally disturbing, especially when pregnancy has proceeded beyond the first trimester. It is not astonishing that in some women such a decision can lead to immediate or late emotional reactions. On the contrary, such sequelae can occur after any major, far-reaching decision in life.

However, it is important to realize that both the difficulties encountered during the decision-making process and the occurrence of psychological sequelae in the aftermath are related to the social acceptance of abortion in the environment of the woman concerned. The best way of minimizing such risks is an open, understanding and sympathetic approach to the problems faced by women with an unwanted pregnancy. In fact this ought to be the normal attitude of any physician towards his or her patients.

Whilst this will remain essential irrespective of the method used, future studies on the merits and hazards of various methodological approaches to the termination of pregnancy may well need to devote more attention to their possible psychological impact than has hitherto been the case.

REFERENCES

1. Zimmerman MK: Passage through abortion: the personal and social reality of women's experiences, pp. 19–31. Praeger, New York, London, 1977.
2. Illsley R and Hall MH: Psychosocial aspects of abortion: a review of issues and needed research. *Bull WHO* 53: 83–106, 1976.
3. David HP: Psychosocial studies of abortion in the United States. In: *Abortion in Psychosocial Perspective: Trends in Transnational Research*. David HP, Friedman HL, van der Tak J, Sevilla MJ (eds), pp. 75–115. Springer, New York, 1978.
4. Adler NE: Emotional responses of women following therapeutic abortion. *Am J Orthopsychiatry* 43: 446–454, 1975.
5. Osofsky JD, Osofsky HJ and Rajan R: Psychological effects of abortion: with emphasis upon immediate reactions and follow-up. In: *The Abortion Experience*, Osofsky HJ and Osofsky JD (eds), pp. 188–205. Hagerstown, MD, 1973.
6. Kaltreider NB: Psychological factors in midtrimester abortion. *Psychiat Med* 4: 132–133, 1973.
7. Athanasiou R, Oppel W, Michelson L. Unger T and Yager M: Psychiatric sequelae to term birth and induced early and late abortion: a longitudinal study. *Fam Plann Perspect* 5: 227–231, 1973.
8. Kerenyi TD, Glascock EL and Horowitz ML: Reasons for delayed abortion: results of 400 interviews. *Am J Obstet Gynecol* 117: 299–311, 1973.
9. Fielding WL, Sachtleben MR, Friedman LM and Friedman EA: Comparison of women seeking early and late abortion. *Am J Obstet Gynecol* 131: 304–310, 1978.

# INDEX